D1029331

Clinical Epidemiology: The Study
of the Outcome of Illness

Monographs in Epidemiology and Biostatistics
edited by Abraham M. Lilienfeld

Monographs in Epidemiology and Biostatistics
Volume 11

Clinical Epidemiology: The Study of the Outcome of Illness

NOEL S. WEISS

New York   Oxford
OXFORD UNIVERSITY PRESS
1986

Oxford University Press

Oxford   New York   Toronto
Delhi   Bombay   Calcutta   Madras   Karachi
Petaling Jaya   Singapore   Hong Kong   Tokyo
Nairobi   Dar es Salaam   Cape Town
Melbourne   Auckland
and associated companies in
Beirut   Berlin   Ibadan   Nicosia

Library of Congress Cataloging-in-Publication Data
Weiss, Noel S., 1943–
Clinical epidemiology.
(Monographs in epidemiology and biostatistics ; v. 11)
Includes bibliographies and index.
1. Epidemiology.   2. Medicine, Clinical.   I. Title.   II. Series.
[DNLM: 1. Biometry.   2. Epidemiologic Methods.   3. Epidemiology.
W1 MO567LT v.11 / WA 950 W431c]
RA652.W45   1986   614.4   85-15503
ISBN 0-19-503718-9

Printing (last digit): 9 8 7 6 5 4 3 2 1

Printed in the United States of America

Preface

This book intends to pull together a number of areas of research that are devoted to measuring and determining the factors that affect the outcome of illness. It gives these areas of research a collective label: clinical epidemiology. This is a term that has been used to mean various things, the most common being epidemiologic research conducted in the "clinic" (or other institution in which health care is provided) by clinicians. In this book, however, the distinction between epidemiologic and clinical epidemiologic research will be made on the basis of the *subject* of the inquiry, that is, the causes versus the consequences of illness.

My goal in writing the book has been to enhance the skills of persons who are conducting or interpreting research that relates to the impact of diagnostic or therapeutic procedures on illness outcome, whether those persons are physicians, nurses, dentists, veterinarians, or other providers of health care. I have assumed that readers will be familiar with such topics as rates and probability, topics that would be covered in an introductory epidemiology or biostatistics course, so the book also may be of benefit to students of epidemiology or biostatistics who are considering work in the clinical setting.

The book begins with a description of the clinical context into which the research findings ought to fit, hence the discussion of decision analysis. Next, there are chapters on the evaluation of diagnostic tests with respect to both their accuracy and their measurable contribution to illness outcome. The discussion of therapy is in two parts—efficacy and safety. The former is sufficiently lengthy to warrant separate chapters for experimental and nonexperimental approaches. The concluding chapter of the book concentrates on the role of studies that measure the natural history of illness. An appendix presents selected statistical methods commonly used in planning and analyzing data from clinical epidemiologic studies.

The book can be read in an armchair, but to get the most out of some sections it would be useful to have a desk, calculator, pencil, and paper. To encourage the active participation of the reader, I have included questions (with answers) at the end of each chapter.

I am grateful to the University of Washington School of Public Health and Community Medicine for providing me the opportunity to develop a course in clinical epidemiology, and to the University of California at Los Angeles School of Public Health for providing the sheltered environment I needed to begin to put the content of that course into the form of a book. Discussions with Drs. Richard Kronmal and Karen Sherman helped me to sharpen my thinking on several of the issues I have chosen to present. Drs. Thomas Koepsell and Nancy Stevens read the entire manuscript; its clarity has been substantially increased as a result of their efforts. My wife and other members of my family have been an unwavering source of support, from well before the conception of this work through the entire period of its gestation.

Seattle, Washington   N.S.W.
May 1985

Contents

Clinical Epidemiology: The Study
of the Outcome of Illness

1 Clinical Epidemiology: What It Is and How It Is Used

Let's say that among your patients is a middle-aged man with intermittent claudication and that his symptoms have been increasing in severity over the last several years. His blood sugar level is normal, but he has a long history of cigarette smoking. The results of the physical examination are normal except for the absence of pulses in the legs. Should he be advised to undergo arteriographic evaluation and an operation for any surgically correctable lesions?

Among the questions that need to be addressed before making such a recommendation are the following: 1. What is the expected progression of symptoms and expected longevity in such a patient in the absence of surgical intervention? 2. To what extent is arteriography capable of (a) identifying remediable lesions, (b) not producing false-positive films, and (c) not producing adverse effects? 3. What is the likelihood (short- and long-term) that surgery can relieve symptoms or prevent progression while at the same time not cause complications? The area of research that attempts to provide answers to these sorts of questions is clinical epidemiology.

Epidemiology per se is the study of variation in the occurrence of disease, and of the reasons for that variation. It first entails making *observations* of individuals (or of populations), for instance, who develops disease and what are the characteristics of the ill or injured individuals that distinguish them from other persons. This process is followed by the formation of *inferences* as to which of these characteristics, or other unmeasured ones, played a role in causing the disease.

Clinical epidemiology is defined here in a parallel way: It is the

3

study of variation in the *outcome* of illness and of the reasons for that variation. The modus operandi is similar as well. First, observations are made as to the fate of ill persons—who recovers, worsens, develops complications, and what characterizes those who have different fates. Second, inferences are made as to the particular characteristics of the patient or his or her care that were responsible for these differences in outcome.

For many conditions, the most important determinants of outcome are diagnostic and therapeutic interventions. Because research in clinical epidemiology attempts to quantify the importance of these interventions relative to others possible or to none at all, the results obtained have direct applications for providers of health care.

To illustrate the questions that epidemiology and clinical epidemiology try to answer, let's return to our patient with claudication. Epidemiologic studies would make observations pertinent to the etiology of the symptom and its underlying pathology: Cigarette smokers and nonsmokers might be contrasted regarding the prevalence of claudication. If this study and others indicated a strong relationship, perhaps one that increased with the amount and recency of smoking, and if nonepidemiologic evidence were compatible with a deleterious effect of cigarette smoking on the peripheral arteries, then an inference of cause and effect could be drawn.

Clinical epidemiology, however, focuses on the consequences of the condition and the care given for it. Thus, observations might be made of untreated patients with claudication regarding the rate of change in symptoms, of other patients undergoing arteriography to determine the prevalence of surgically correctable lesions, and of still others who undergo surgery to assess the change in symptoms and/or physical signs. These studies would lead to inferences as to the role of surgery in achieving the intended purpose: To what extent was there improvement of symptoms and signs in patients who underwent these procedures? To what extent could any favorable outcomes be attributed to spontaneous regression of disease, or to selection for surgical therapy of patients destined to have favorable outcomes? If arteriography/surgery did produce improvements, what proportion of the patients undergoing arteriography was helped? By how much? Quantitative answers are necessary, for they will have to be balanced against the costs and hazards of arteriography and surgery (see below).

Though the term illness is part of the definition of clinical epidemiology, no attempt will be made to define it in any precise way. "Illness" is used here in a far broader sense than is "disease," which often refers to a particular set of anatomic or physiologic abnormalities. Illness may, for example, denote only a symptom that causes a patient to seek care, or to a physical sign detected by a provider of care. Since a large part of the utility of research in clinical epidemiology lies in its evaluation of the work of providers of health care, illness here will refer to any reason people have for seeking the services of such a provider. The methods of clinical epidemiology operate in the same fashion, whether they are applied to persons seeking care for health maintenance, for a specific symptom or sign, or for a disease.

WAYS IN WHICH CLINICAL EPIDEMIOLOGY IS PUT TO USE: DECISION MAKING

Virtually everything we can do for a patient has a "cost" attached to it. Costs can be measured in terms of labor and/or materials expended for the patient's care, such as those involved in taking a medical history, administering diagnostic roentgenography, or synthesizing and marketing a drug. A second cost relates to the deleterious effects on the patient's well-being of some aspects of the care provided. A barium enema will result in radiation exposure in all patients, cause temporary discomfort in most of them, and in rare instances lead to more serious consequences (e.g., bowel perforation). Digitalis will cause side effects in many patients, some minor (e.g., nausea) and some potentially severe (e.g., cardiac arrhythmias).

Ideally, no diagnostic or therapeutic measure should be undertaken unless its expected benefits to the patient exceed its expected costs. In most situations, an estimate of the relative magnitude of benefits and costs is easily made. In a patient with pneumococcal pneumonia, the therapeutic benefit of penicillin clearly outweighs the possibility of anaphylaxis (or other adverse effect) and the dollar cost of the drug. In an 85-year-old patient with angina, the various costs of coronary angiography and coronary artery bypass surgery almost always will outweigh the expected benefits in terms of symptom relief or (perhaps) increased longevity.

However, a number of situations confront the provider of care in which there appears to exist a near balance of benefits and costs.

For example, at present it is not clear to many providers whether, in order to detect cancer of the large bowel at an early stage, they should examine feces for occult blood using the Hemoccult test in asymptomatic, previously unscreened adult patients. In favor of the decision to use the test is the fact that some patients with undiagnosed cancer of this type who would have died of it will, instead, through treatment of tumors found at an early stage, be cured. Arguing against the use of the Hemoccult test in these patients is the cost of the test itself and the cost of evaluating further persons whose tests are positive but who do not have cancer.

In situations like this, one means of structuring the available information in order to guide the provider's use of diagnostic and therapeutic measures is *decision analysis.* The way in which decision analysis proceeds is illustrated in Figure 1-1. For purposes of this example it will be assumed that (a) the prevalence of cancer of the large bowel in this patient group is 2 per 1,000 and that, in the absence of Hemoccult testing, one-half of those with the cancer will die within the next 3 years; (b) 2% of those tested will be "positive," but among them 92% will be falsely positive (in most asymptomatic persons with blood in their stool, the source of the blood is not a malignancy of the large bowel); (c) a few people (0.04%) will test negative but will actually have the cancer; (d) the 3-year mortality in screened persons with cancer is only 40%, and that of persons without cancer is 2% (with or without screening); (e) other than cost, there are no negative attributes of Hemoccult testing (this will not necessarily be the case for other screening and diagnostic tests, the morbidity of which would have to be incorporated into the "decision tree").

The process of weighing the two alternatives (screen or not screen) begins by enumerating every possible category of patient, first of those who undergo testing and then of patients who do not. (For simplicity, the example described in Figure 1-1 ignores many important outcomes, primarily those relating to morbidity from colorectal cancer and its treatment.) Thus, the top "branch" in Figure 1-1 refers to patients who were screened, had a positive Hemoccult test, were found on further testing to have colorectal cancer, and who, despite the screening, died during the next 3 years.

Second, the proportion of patients in each category is estimated by multiplying together all of the probabilities of the "steps" that define the category. For example, the proportion of screened individuals found to be positive, who have colorectal cancer, and who

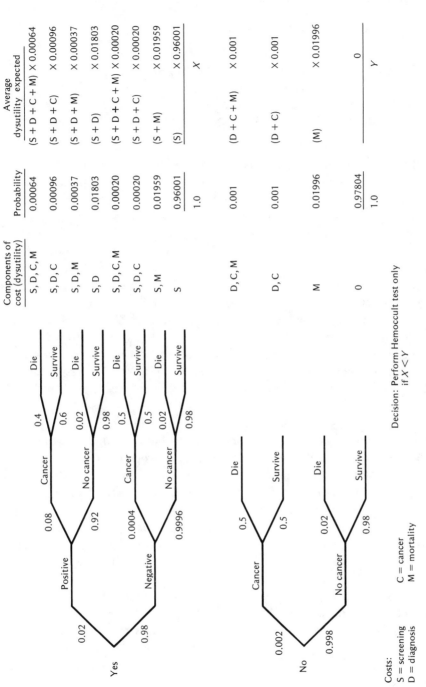

Figure 1-1. Decision tree for performing the Hemoccult test in asymptomatic patients.

	Components of cost (dysutility)	Probability	Average dysutility expected
Die	S, D, C, M	0.00064	(S + D + C + M) × 0.00064
Survive	S, D, C	0.00096	(S + D + C) × 0.00096
Die	S, D, M	0.00037	(S + D + M) × 0.00037
Survive	S, D	0.01803	(S + D) × 0.01803
Die	S, D, C, M	0.00020	(S + D + C + M) × 0.00020
Survive	S, D, C	0.00020	(S + D + C) × 0.00020
Die	S, M	0.01959	(S + M) × 0.01959
Survive	S	0.96001	(S) × 0.96001
		1.0	X
Die	D, C, M	0.001	(D + C + M) × 0.001
Survive	D, C	0.001	(D + C) × 0.001
Die	M	0.01996	(M) × 0.01996
Survive	0	0.97804	0
		1.0	Y

Costs:
S = screening   C = cancer
D = diagnosis   M = mortality

Decision: Perform Hemoccult test only
if $X < Y$

7

die of the cancer within 3 years is equal to:

0.02	(proportion screened as positive)
× 0.08	(proportion of these patients who have cancer)
× 0.4	(proportion of cancer patients screened as positive
0.0064	who die within 3 years)

Third, a weight or value is assigned to each possible category. These values are the sums of the costs—monetary, physical, and emotional—of the disease and the testing and treatment of it. These values are all negative, for the occurrence of cancer of the large bowel exerts a negative influence on the population's health; hence the terms costs and dysutilities used in Figure 1-1 and hereafter. In question is whether or not the expenditure of some of the population's resources, for instance, on screening, will diminish this negative influence.

Fourth, the proportion of patients in each category is multiplied by the negative value attached to that category. Finally, the sum of these products ("average dysutility expected") for persons undergoing Hemoccult testing (X) is compared with the corresponding sum for persons not tested (Y). If $X < Y$, then testing should be recommended.

Often there is uncertainty as to the probability with which some of the events occur, for instance, the probability of death among screened and unscreened persons with colorectal cancer, or as to the size of the dysutility associated with a particular category of patient (see below). A useful feature of decision analysis is that, once the structures of the decision trees have been developed, the extent to which the decision is affected by changes in the probabilities of the various outcomes or in the particular set of dysutilities chosen can be determined. This process of determining if the decision is influenced by changes in the input information is called "sensitivity analysis." It allows the decision-maker to determine how solid his or her choice is, despite imprecise knowledge.

This book is devoted to describing the means by which one measures the probability of occurrence of the steps that define each category of patient outcome, but as for the measurement of the dysutilities, a few paragraphs here must do. Certainly, some of the dysutilities are easy to estimate accurately, for example, the dollar cost of the Hemoccult test and of the procedures needed to secure a diagnosis. The impact of having the cancer is harder to quantify.

The average cost of treatment can be determined, but what of the physical and psychological effects? And what is the "cost" of death? And, if we are to complete the decision analysis, how can we put these dollar, illness, and death dysutilities in the same units?

As difficult as the task is, in order for providers to make rational decisions regarding the delivery of health care—whether or not they employ decision analysis in a formal way—it is necessary that they weigh the various negative events on a common scale. Most often, the scale is a monetary one. The idea of assigning a certain monetary value to health or to a human life is an unappealing one to most of us, and rarely is anyone in a position to knowingly cause loss of health or life in a specific individual by failing to make a dollar expenditure. Nonetheless, society chooses to allocate only so many of its dollars for reducing the probability of illness and death among its members. We are willing to pay so much, but not more, for road safety, for example. It is probable that additional highway dividers or railroad bridges would prevent some injuries and an occasional accidental traffic death, but in many instances we are unable to "afford" them. Or, perhaps, we may believe that installation of a highly trained, rapid-response, emergency medical service in a town of 10,000 persons could lead to the survival of one person who develops cardiac arrest each year, but it is likely that in many towns of this size, the expense of operating such a program is beyond what the populace is willing to pay.

Since society is responsible for the overwhelming majority of expenditures for health care, the wishes of society should play the major role in determining whether or not individual health care expenses are met as well. Though a provider of health care is committed to doing everything possible to promote a patient's health, the range of what is possible should be delineated by those who will pay the bill. Thus, there are instances in which a health care provider, conscious of society's needs, actually will make recommendations or take actions that fall short of those that he or she would implement if resources for health care were unlimited. Such a provider realizes that these resources *are* limited—what is consumed for one purpose is not available for others. The goal of the health care provider, then, is to use these finite resources in the most efficient way. For example, a provider might be willing to do a Pap smear every 3 years rather than more frequently in women already screened several times as negative, not because this approach is adequate to prevent all mortality from cervical cancer in such patients but because it is a reasonably inexpensive way to prevent *most* of it.

Example. In patients with acute chest pain, several clinical characteristics have been identified that are correlated with the presence of myocardial infarction. A group of investigators (Fineberg et al., 1984) attempted to assess the economic and health implications of two types of acute care in patients with chest pain who are in a "low" risk group (probability of myocardial infarction less than 1 in 20): (a) admission to a coronary care unit versus (b) admission to an "intermediate" care unit (i.e., one that would permit electrocardiographic monitoring and the administration of prophylactic lidocaine but not intensive nursing care). They estimated that there would be a small excess of deaths from ventricular fibrillation and complete heart block in the group placed in intermediate care. Nonetheless, they concluded that "patients who have a low risk for myocardial infarction would be appropriate candidates for admission to an 'intermediate' care unit, since the provision of the facilities of a coronary care unit to all low risk patients would cost an estimated additional $2 million per life saved."

If we are (reluctantly) willing to assign costs to the loss of health and human life, how do we go about deciding what these costs should be? To catalog the techniques that have been devised to do this is beyond the scope of this book, so an example will suffice: One could visit a sample of residents in the hypothetical town mentioned earlier, describe the emergency medical service and its expected benefits (in terms of lives saved), and ask how much each resident would be willing to add to the annual town tax to enable such a service to be established. The average dollar figure obtained in the sample, multiplied by the number of persons in the town, divided by the number of lives saved per year (1.0 in this example) gives an estimate of how much the townspeople would be willing to spend in the effort to prevent the loss of one life.

This and other methods of estimating the "cost" of a human life clearly are not going to be as precise as those that estimate screening costs, hospitalization costs, and so on. For this reason, it is particularly important to determine how sensitive any decision is to changes over a plausibly wide range of such costs.

It is possible to further embellish this process by incorporating the fact that, when forced to make the choice, most of us would save the life of (a) a 30-year-old rather than an 80-year-old, or (b) someone with no disability rather than a quadriplegic. What emerges from this refinement is a comparison not of dollars per life saved but rather of dollars per *quality-adjusted years* of life saved. Embellished or not, the basic idea is that in making decisions about expenditures that could prevent mortality or morbidity—whether such decisions relate to highway design, emergency medical services, or clinical practice—the question of the cost of that prevention is always considered, at least implicitly.

In summary, the process of decision analysis requires two ingredients: the "cost" associated with each category of patient outcome, either a direct dollar expenditure or a physical manifestation (illness, death) that is translated into a monetary equivalent, and the likelihood of each outcome. Estimating the latter is the business of clinical epidemiology, and it involves estimating first the probabilities at each "branch" of the decision tree. These then are multiplied together to arrive at an estimate of the overall likelihood. So, in attempting to determine if it is desirable to perform testing for fecal occult blood (Figure 1-1) it is necessary to estimate the probability of (a) test positivity, (b) positively and negatively testing persons having cancer of the large bowel, and (c) the survival of persons with cancer conditional on being tested and (if so) on the test results. Clinical epidemiologic studies are those that gather data from which these probabilities can be assessed. The resulting probabilities then can be used to make inferences regarding (a) the usefulness of a diagnostic or screening test, (b) the efficacy or safety of a therapeutic measure, and (c) the likelihood or speed with which progression or complications occur in persons with a given condition ("natural history"). These topics are dealt with, in turn, in the rest of this book.

QUESTIONS, CHAPTER 1

1-1. You are the head of a general surgical unit. For patients who have undergone cholecystectomy, the unit's policy has been to require a minimum of 10 postoperative days of hospitalization. However, you are aware that others have developed a policy of hospital discharge as soon as a patient meets a number of preset clinical criteria (e.g., no requirement for parenteral analgesics or nursing care for eating and dressing, return of urinary and bowel function, good wound healing), irrespective of duration of postoperative stay. You mention the issue to your hospital administrator, who encourages you to look further into this potential cost-saving approach.

You come upon in the literature a report of a randomized controlled trial that has tested these two postoperative strategies ("fixed" vs. flexible" stay) in 100 patients (Simpson et al., 1977). The results are summarized below:

	Patient group:	
	"Fixed" post-op stay ($n = 47$)	"Flexible" post-op stay ($n = 53$)
Mean duration of post-op stay (days)	9.7	7.6
No. of hospital readmissions	0	0
No. of post-op deaths	0	0
No. with need for outpatient services within 3 weeks of surgery	16 (34%)	29 (55%)

While the policy of flexible discharge based on fulfillment of clinical criteria led to a 2-day reduction in length of hospital stay, it also led to an increase in utilization of outpatient services. In addition, it is possible that the frequency of hospital readmission (and possibly of late postoperative mortality) might be increased in the flexible discharge group, but that in a study of only 100 patients such an increase might not have been detectable.

To sort out these issues in a systematic way, you perform an elementary decision analysis. For the fixed-stay group, you construct the following decision tree:

"Fixed" post-op stay

			Dysutilities ($):				
			9.7 inpatient days	Readmission	Death	Outpatient services	Total
Readmission 0.05	Died		2,910	2,000	200,000	0	
0.01 0.95	Survived		2,910	2,000	0	0	
0.99 No readmission 0.34	Outpatient services needed		2,910	0	0	100	
0.66	No outpatient services needed		2,910	0	0	0	‗‗‗

In setting up the tree you make a guess that some of these patients (say, 1%) will require readmission, and that 5% of those readmitted will die as a complication of surgery. (For simplicity, you assume that no one requiring readmission will also require outpatient services and that no one who is not readmitted will die of these complications.) Your administrator tells you that 1 postoperative day in the hospital costs about $300, and you estimate a readmission to last 5 days at $400 per day. From the literature you find an estimated "value" for a human life that is on the high side ($200,000) and guess that outpatient costs would be around $100.

What is the total average postoperative cost associated with this fixed-stay policy?

1-2. Construct a similar decision tree for a flexible-stay policy. Calculate the total average postoperative cost associated with this policy, assuming that the possibility of readmission is higher than that under the fixed-stay policy by a factor of (a) 1.1, (b) 2, or (c) 5. (Assume that among those readmitted, the probability of death remains the same as under the fixed-stay policy, i.e., 5%.) Based on this analysis, which of the two policies should you adopt?

ANSWERS

1-1. $3,063.66

1-2.   *"Flexible" post-op stay*

			Dysutilities ($):			
		7.6 inpatient days	Readmis- sion	Death	Outpatient services	Total
	Died	2,280	2000	200,000	0	112.35
0.05 Readmission						
0.95 Survived		2,280	2000	0	0	44.73
Outpatient services needed		2,280	0	0	100	1294.60
0.55						
No readmission						
No outpatient services						
0.45 needed		2,280	0	0	0	1041.71
						2466.40

0.011

0.989

Probability of readmission	Average post-op cost of flexible-stay policy
0.011	$2,466.40
0.020	$2,573.90
0.050	$2,932.25

Even under the extreme assumption of a fivefold increase in the occurrence of complications leading to readmission and death, the average postoperative cost per case under the flexible-stay policy is less than that ($3,063.66) under the fixed-stay policy. Thus, based on the factors considered here, it would be prudent to switch to the flexible-stay policy for patients recovering from cholecystectomy.

REFERENCES

Fineberg HV, Scadden D, Goldman L: Care of patients with a low probability of acute myocardial infarction: Cost effectiveness of alternatives to coronary-care-unit admission. *N Engl J Med* 1984; 310:1301–1307.

Simpson JEP, Cox AG, Meade TW, et al: "Right" stay in hospital after surgery: Randomised controlled trial. *Br Med J* 1977; 1:1514–1516.

2 Diagnostic and Screening Tests: What Information Is Needed Before Developing a Policy for Their Use?

MEASURING THE VALIDITY OF A TEST

When you choose to buy information in the form of the results of diagnostic or screening tests, you do so because you believe that the value of the information exceeds its price. The value of a test result depends both on its accuracy and on how important the result is in leading to action(s) that bear on the individual's well-being. (Assessing the latter is the subject of Chapter 3.)

The accuracy of a test depends, in turn, on its reliability—the degree to which repeated measurements give the same result—and its validity—the degree to which it measures what it intends to. The following exercise introduces some measures of test validity:

Example. Two physicians have attempted to develop clinical criteria to predict, among patients who have had head trauma, which ones are helped by an x-ray examination of the skull. Some of the criteria they thought might be important were duration of unconsciousness, external wounds of the head, and positive neurologic findings. They tested their criteria in 1,500 patients who were seen in a hospital emergency room and who underwent skull roentgenography, classifying each patient as "positive" or "negative" with regard to the suspected probability of having a skull fracture (Bell and Loop, 1971). The results were as follows (for purposes of this example it is assumed that a skull x-ray film measures perfectly the presence or absence of skull fracture):

Screening criteria:

		Positive	Negative	
Skull fracture:	Yes	92	1	93
	No	973	434	1,407
		1,065	435	1,500

The accuracy of the clinical criteria (the "test") could be described in terms of the degree to which persons with and without the condition under study (skull fracture) are correctly categorized. So, the percentage of persons with a fracture who tested positive by the clinical criteria—the "sensitivity" of the criteria—was $92/93 \times 100 = 98.9\%$. The percentage of persons without a fracture who were correctly categorized as negative by the criteria—the "specificity"—was $434/1,407 \times 100 = 30.8\%$.

Alternatively, the accuracy of the criteria could be stated as the extent to which being categorized as positive or negative actually predicts the presence of a fracture. In this example, the percentage of persons who were deemed clinically positive and who were found to have a fracture—the predictive value of a positive test (PV+)—was $92/1,065 \times 100 = 8.6\%$. The percentage who were clinically negative and who truly had no fracture—the predictive value of a negative test (PV−)—was $434/435 \times 100 = 99.8\%$. These measures are summarized in Table 2-1.

ESTIMATION OF PREDICTIVE VALUE UNDER VARIOUS SAMPLING SCHEMES

Obviously, having an understanding of the validity of the clinical criteria in predicting the presence of a skull fracture is only the first step in reaching a decision as to whether these criteria should be used in managing patients with head trauma. It is also necessary to take into account the relevant costs—of applying the criteria to individual patients, of performing skull roentgenography, and of the morbidity and mortality from fracture—before an informed decision can be made. An analysis of the virtues of the two options, skull x-ray tests only for clinically positive patients versus skull x-ray tests for all, is presented in Figure 2-1.

From Figure 2-1 it can be seen that two of the measures of test accuracy that were calculated earlier, the predictive values of a positive and negative test (92/1,065 and 434/435, respectively), were entered directly into the decision trees. These are the measures that we are interested in estimating with particular accuracy from studies that evaluate the validity of a test. So, it is necessary to be aware of some commonly used study designs from which it is not possible to calculate directly PV+ and/or PV−.

(1) For instance, a study of the accuracy of screening criteria for skull fracture might compare the known fracture cases with a sample of noncases, rather than with the entire fracture-free group with

Table 2-1. Measures of the Accuracy of a Diagnostic Test

	General Test Criterion:				*Example* Test criterion:		
	Positive	Negative			Positive	Negative	
Reference criterion	a	b	a + b	Fracture	92	1	93
	c	d	c + d	No fracture	973	434	1,407
	a + c	b + d	n		1,065	435	1,500

Term	General	Example	Definition
a. Sensitivity	a/(a + b)	92/93	Proportion of those with the condition who have a positive test
b. Specificity	d/(c + d)	434/1,407	Proportion of those without the condition who have a negative test
c. Predictive value of a positive test (PV+)	a/(a + c)^a	92/1,065	Proportion of those with a positive test who have the condition
d. Predictive value of a negative test (PV−)	d/(b + d)^a	434/435	Proportion of those with a negative test who do not have the condition

[a]Only meaningful if (a + b)/n represents the actual proportion of true-positives in the relevant population. If this condition does not hold, the test's sensitivity and specificity can be used to estimate the predictive values (see p. 18).

head trauma. In the following example, equal numbers of noncases and cases have been chosen. If the proportion of screened-positive and screened-negative patients among noncases mirrors that of the total population of noncases [(973/1,407) × 93 = 64 falling in the positive group], the data would appear as follows:

Screening criteria:

		Positive	Negative	
	Yes	92	1	93
Skull fracture:				
	No	64	29	93
		156	30	

Clearly, it would be incorrect to calculate PV+ as 92/156 or PV− as 29/30. These calculations are strongly affected by the relative number of persons in the groups with and without fracture, and, in this example, these numbers have been arbitrarily set (one control per one fracture case). However, the sensitivity and specificity of the screening criteria can be accurately determined (each is calculated

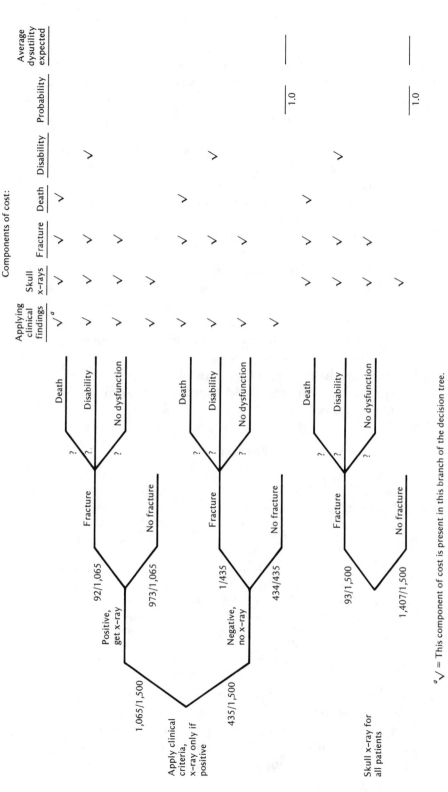

Figure 2-1. Clinical findings as criteria for obtaining skull x-rays.

[a] = This component of cost is present in this branch of the decision tree.

within the group of fracture cases and noncases, respectively), and if the frequency of the condition that is being screened can be estimated, both predictive values can be estimated as well. The most straightforward way of doing this is as follows:

1. Pick, arbitrarily, a number representing the size of the total group that might be tested (or screened). Let's say you choose 10,000.
2. Multiply this number by the prevalence of the condition for which testing (or screening) is being performed. Let's say you happen to know that the prevalence of skull fracture in patients seeking care for head trauma is 6.2% (i.e., the prevalence in the full study of 1,500 patients). Thus, of the 10,000 patients, 620 would have a fracture and 9,380 would not.
3a. Multiply the number of patients with the condition by the sensitivity of the test to determine the number of true-positives.
3b. Multiply the number of patients without the condition by the specificity of the test to determine the number of true-negatives. The resulting table should look like this:

Clinical criteria:

Skull fracture	Positive	Negative	
Yes	$620 \times 92/93 = 613$	b	620
No	c	$9,380 \times 29/93 = 2,925$	9,380
			10,000

4. By subtraction, determine the number of false-negatives and false-positives. In this example, there would be 7 false-negatives ($620 - 613$) and 6,455 false-positives ($9,380 - 2,925$).
5. Calculate the PV+ and PV− from the numbers in the table:

$$PV+ = 613/(613 + 6,455) = 8.7\%$$
$$PV- = 2,925/(2,925 + 7) = 99.8\%$$

These values are identical (save for errors due to rounding) to those calculated from the entire 1,500 patients with head trauma.

Thus, the accurate estimation of PV+ and PV− requires either (a) the use of a study population in which the frequency of the condition being tested for approximates that of the population in which the results are to be applied or (b) a knowledge of the frequency of the condition in the population in which the results are to be applied. These requirements underscore the influence of the frequency of the condition in the population being tested on the size of the predictive values and, ultimately, the influence of the frequency on the usefulness of the test in question. If a condition is uncommon, even a test that is highly sensitive and specific may produce a PV+ that is quite low. The following table, constructed for a test with both sensitivity and specificity of 97%, illustrates this phenomenon:

Proportion of the tested population with the condition	PV+	PV−
0.1	0.782	0.997
0.01	0.246	0.9997
0.001	0.031	0.99997
0.0001	0.003	0.999997

In this example, only when 10% of the persons receiving the test have the condition is PV+ greater than 0.5. For a frequency of 1/1,000 or less, PV+ is so low (≤ 0.031) that the test would probably not be useful for clinical or public health purposes. (It would be useful only if the cost of a false-positive were exceedingly small compared with the benefit of identifying a true-positive.) The PV− gradually approaches 1.0 with decreasing disease frequency, and, compared with the PV+, exhibits little variation. However, keep in mind that even small changes in the PV− may be crucial in deciding whether or not a test should be used. For example, one reason that screening criteria for skull roentgenography have been adopted by many providers of care is a high value for PV−; only a very small proportion of clinically "negative" persons have fractures. If that proportion were to increase by even a small amount, many of these providers, concerned about the number of persons who test falsely negative and the consequences to them, might choose to abandon these criteria and administer x-rays to all patients with head trauma.

(2) The previous example dealt with studies in which the proportions of person with and without the condition for which testing was done (e.g., skull fracture) did not reflect those of the population in which the results were to be applied (e.g., patients with head trauma admitted to an emergency room). Conversely, there are situations in which the proportions of study subjects who do and do not receive the test do not reflect those of the population in which the

results are to be applied. For instance, suppose you are analyzing data from another hospital emergency room in which there were the same number of clinically positive patients as in the example in Table 2-1, but patients with mild head trauma also came for evaluation. Instead of the ratio of clinically positive to negative cases of 1,065/435 encountered in that example, the ratio now is 1,065/1,305. Assuming that the frequency of fracture among these 870 additional clinically negative cases were the same as among the original 435, the data relating the clinical screening criteria to fracture occurrence would look like this:

Screening criteria:

Positive Negative

		Positive	Negative	
Skull fracture:	Yes	92	3	95
	No	973	1,302	2,275
		1,065	1,305	2,370

The predictive values would be calculated as before (PV+ = 92/1,065 = 0.086; PV− = 1,302/1,305 = 0.998). Apparently all that has changed are the proportions of clinically positive and clinically negative patients.

But there is a possible pitfall here. Among persons with head trauma who are "negative" according to the clinical criteria decided upon by the investigators, there will be a spectrum of severity. Those with the least trauma will be the least likely to go to the emergency room and also the least likely to have skull fractures. So, of the 870 additional clinically negative patients with head trauma coming to the second emergency room there may be *no* additional patients with fracture, rather than the two expected. If this were true, not only the sensitivity and specificity but the PV− would be affected: PV− would be 1,303/1,304 = 0.9992, a value higher than that obtained for the first emergency room, where the PV− was 434/435 = 0.9977. (The PV+ will be unaffected by all of this, for it is based only on results in clinically positive individuals.) Thus, in order for a PV− observed in a study population to be applied in a valid way in a particular reference population, it is necessary to consider the similarity of the two populations with respect to the types of patients that did and did not receive the test.

(3) A situation in which neither PV+ nor PV− can be estimated accurately is one in which subjects with a condition or illness are not typical of ill subjects for whom the test is intended, with respect to the likelihood of a positive test result. For example, if the Hemoccult test were administered to symptomatic persons with colorectal cancer, rather than to the asymptomatic population for whom it is meant to be administered for screening purposes, the calculated sensitivity would almost certainly be artificially high. It is probable that symptomatic patients have a relatively more advanced condition and would have a higher probability of having blood in their stool. Thus, even though the specificity of the Hemoccult test could be assessed accurately in this design—specificity is based solely on the results in noncases—the PV+ and PV− would be falsely high.

SINGLE MEASURES OF TEST VALIDITY

Some have fallen prey to the temptation to summarize the assessment of the validity of a test with a single figure. Most commonly, this is the percentage of patients correctly classified by the test. [This measure has been termed the "efficiency" of a test (Galen and Gambino, 1975)]. Using the skull fracture example, this percentage would be

$$\frac{\text{true-positives} + \text{true-negatives}}{\text{total patients}} \times 100 = \frac{92 + 434}{1,500} \times 100 = 35.1\%$$

Summary measures, such as the "percent correctly classified," should be avoided for at least two reasons. First, they do not fit into the decision-making process regarding the use of the test, as do the positive and negative predictive values. Second, they can give misleading results. For example, consider a test with a sensitivity of zero and a specificity of 100%, that is, a test that labels every subject as not having the condition. In the skull fracture example, this completely valueless test would still correctly classify 93.8% {[(0 + 1,407)/1,500] × 100} of the subjects, a value far higher than could be obtained using the clinical criteria (35.1%).

OTHER INFORMATION NEEDED TO COMPLETE
THE DECISION ANALYSIS

So far, we have discussed only the accuracy of a diagnostic or screening test and nothing of the implications of patients being correctly or incorrectly identified as having the condition in question. Data on these implications are usually more difficult to come by, and it is often the case that "holes" in the data must be filled in by good guesses:

A British study (Royal College of Radiologists, 1981) systematically obtained clinical data and roentgenographic results for 5,850 consecutive patients seen at any of nine emergency rooms for head trauma and who received skull x-ray tests. On the basis of criteria similar to those described earlier, patients were classified as being clinically positive or negative before results of the skull x-ray tests and the subsequent course of events were known. The initial clinical status was then related to the roentgenographic diagnosis and to the occurrence of intracranial hematoma and its associated mortality. The following results were obtained:

	n	
Clinically positive patients	2,522	
Skull fracture	99	
(intracranial hematoma)		6 (3 deaths)
No skull fracture	2,423	
(intracranial hematoma)		1 (0 deaths)
Clinically negative patients	3,328	
Skull fracture	23	
(intracranial hematoma)		1 (0 deaths)
No skull fracture	3,305	
(intracranial hematoma)		0

Figures 2.2 and 2.3 are a pair of decision trees that elaborate the components of the choice to employ criteria as a basis for obtaining skull x-ray films in patients with head trauma. Added to the trees used earlier are "limbs" that deal with the consequences of trauma (for purposes of simplicity they are restricted to intracranial hematoma and its associated mortality).

We can calculate most of the probabilities (Figures 2.2 and 2.3), assuming the following: (a) In the absence of an intracranial hematoma, the probability of death from head trauma is zero. (b) Awareness of the presence of a skull fracture does not result in action that can prevent the occurrence of intracranial hematoma. Rather, such awareness enables the rapid diagnosis and treatment of persons with hematoma and reduces the associated case-fatality.

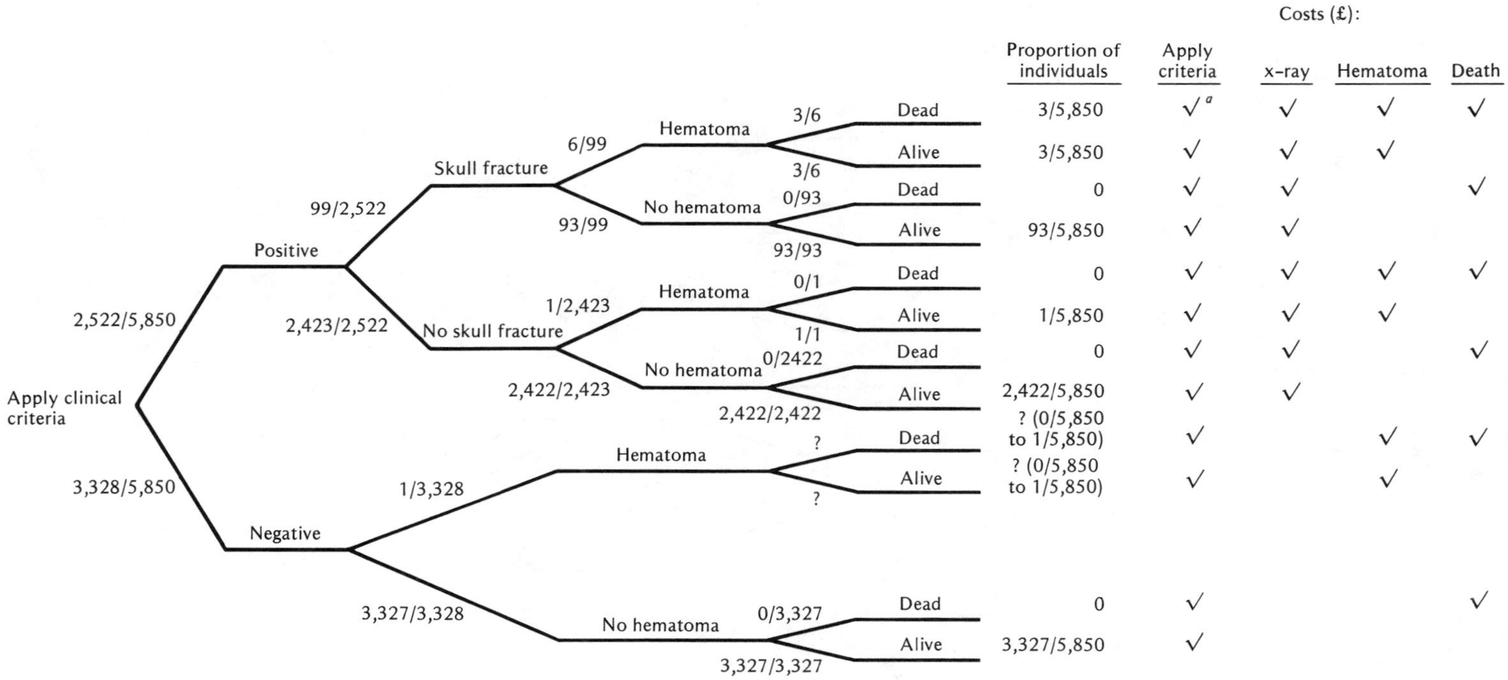

Costs (£):

Proportion of individuals	Apply criteria[a]	x-ray	Hematoma	Death
3/5,850	✓	✓	✓	✓
3/5,850	✓	✓	✓	
0	✓	✓		✓
93/5,850	✓	✓		
0	✓	✓		✓
1/5,850	✓	✓	✓	✓
0	✓	✓	✓	
2,422/5,850	✓	✓		
? (0/5,850 to 1/5,850)	✓	✓	✓	✓
? (0/5,850 to 1/5,850)	✓	✓	✓	
0	✓			✓
3,327/5,850	✓			

Decision tree branches:

Apply clinical criteria

Positive 2,522/5,850
- Skull fracture 99/2,522
  - Hematoma 6/99
    - Dead 3/6
    - Alive 3/6
  - No hematoma 93/99
    - Dead 0/93
    - Alive 93/93
- No skull fracture 2,423/2,522
  - Hematoma 1/2,423
    - Dead 0/1
    - Alive 1/1
  - No hematoma 2,422/2,423
    - Dead 0/2422
    - Alive 2,422/2,422

Negative 3,328/5,850
- Hematoma 1/3,328
  - Dead ?
  - Alive ?
- No hematoma 3,327/3,328
  - Dead 0/3,327
  - Alive 3,327/3,327

[a]✓ = This component of cost is present in this branch of the decision tree.

Figure 2-2. Clinical findings as criteria for obtaining skull x-rays.

23

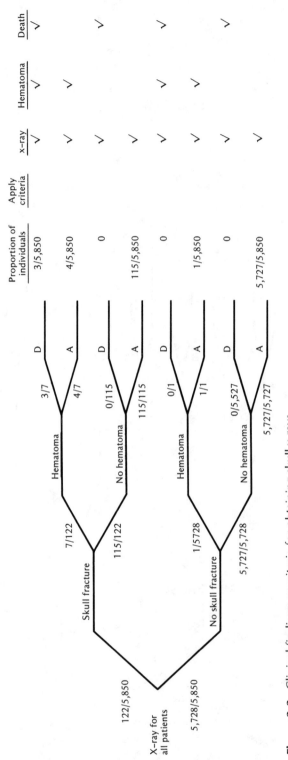

Figure 2-3. Clinical findings as criteria for obtaining skull x-rays.

In broad terms, there are also four possible "costs" associated with this group of patients, those related to applying the criteria, obtaining an x-ray film, intracranial hematoma, and death. The categories of patients in which one or more of these applies are indicated in Figures 2.2 and 2.3.

Based on the information provided, we are able to assign probabilities to all but one of the possible occurrences that we have allowed for. The only uncertainty (apart from sampling error, which for many of these estimates is admittedly great) lies in the group of persons who are clinically negative and do not undergo skull x-ray tests. While we can estimate that there would be one such person (of 5,850 with head trauma) who would develop an intracranial hematoma, we do not have any data on which to base a prognosis, since every person studied had the benefit of a skull x-ray examination. So, since the most important reservations we might have about adopting the clinical criteria are due to worries about the fate of persons in just this category, what have we accomplished?

We will attempt to answer this question by using the information we have regarding probabilities, and by making estimates and educated guesses for the remaining portions of the decisions trees. The goal is to arrive at a series of comparison of the two options (roentgenography for all vs. roentgenography for only those who are clinically positive) over a range of plausible values for the unknown quantities. So let's assume that in Britain a skull x-ray test costs £9 and the medical costs due to morbidity from intracranial hematoma are established at £1,000. Table 2-2 presents estimates as to how the cost (of the head trauma that has been sustained by these 5,850 individuals) would be influenced by the diagnostic strategy (clinical criteria vs. skull x-ray tests for all patients) and by varying assumptions regarding the following: (a) case-fatality for persons who are

Table 2-2. Costs of Head Trauma

| Case-fatality rate[a] | Component of cost (£) | | | Overall cost (£) | |
	Application of clinical criteria	Fatality		Use clinical criteria	x-ray test for all
10%	1	50,000		32.74	36.01
50%	1	50,000		36.16	36.01
10%	1	100,000		59.24	61.65
50%	1	100,000		66.08	61.65
10%	0.5	100,000		58.74	61.65
50%	0.5	100,000		65.58	61.65

[a]In clinically negative persons with an intracranial hematoma.

clinically negative yet have an intracran[...] (b) cost of applying the clinical criteria— a fatality—50,000 or £100,000.

In this example, if the case-fatality i[...] cranial hematoma but who were clinica[...] undergo skull roentgenography) were [...] head trauma places on society would [...] apply the criteria than to request x-r[...] head trauma. On the other hand, if [...] were 50%, ordering x-ray films for al[...] be the better choice with respect to th[...] ments can be made nearly equally wel[...] estimated for the application of the cl[...] That is, the decision is relatively ins[...] costs, within the given range. (Even if it is argued that there is no cost associated with employing the clinical criteria—i.e., that the history and physical findings constituting the criteria are obtained in the normal course of patient care—if a fatality were negatively valued at £100,000, then the direction of the comparison would be unchanged.)

In this example, the range of uncertainty examined for the case-fatality rate was 10% versus 50%, a relatively wider range than that for the various costs. The use of the high or the low value would have a bearing on the decision to use or not use the clinical criteria. Perhaps you (or persons knowledgeable in this area with whom you have discussed the issue) feel that the case-fatality is likely to be much closer to 10% than to 50%. You may reason that if, despite an intracranial hematoma, the patient has no neurological signs or symptoms to suggest such pathology, then his or her chances for survival should be good. In this case, you could, with some confidence, decide to adopt the clinical criteria as a guide for ordering skull x-ray films in subsequent patients with head trauma. If, on the other hand, you have reason to believe that the value of 50% is closer to the truth, you would adopt the opposite policy. Finally, if the two values seem equally plausible, you would not be able to make the decision on a "rational" basis from available data.

If the latter is the case—the analyses you have performed have failed to resolve the issue—then there has nonetheless been a purpose served by having completed this exercise. For it is now apparent that it will be important to obtain more precise knowledge of the case-fatality in asymptomatic intracranial hematoma cases that are not diagnosed initially because skull x-ray films were not obtained. In contrast, it will be less important to estimate more precisely the costs associated with categorizing a patient on the basis of clinical criteria, or the costs that society ascribes to a premature fatality. This formalization of the question has pointed out the direction for the most relevant future research.

In summary, several issues need to be considered when trying to determine if, in a group of patients with defined characteristics, the benefits of administering a test exceed the costs. For most tests these issues are straightforward and a decision to use (or not use) the test can be made easily.

When the "right" decision is not apparent, however, formalization of the decision-making process can be useful. After structuring the outcomes that could occur subsequent to testing or not testing, it is necessary to assemble information regarding (a) the accuracy of the test, (b) the frequency of the condition(s) for which testing is being considered, (c) the degree to which detection *at that time* can reduce the likelihood or severity of consequences of the condition, and (d) the "costs" of the test, of whatever misclassification might ensue, and of the consequences of the condition that one is seeking to prevent. The degree to which accurate estimates can be obtained for these items will vary, and for some it will be possible only to specify a range within which the true value is likely to lie. Thus, when performing the decision analysis it may be necessary to conduct sensitivity testing, that is, to evaluate the decision over a range of values assigned to some or all of the items.

When the analysis is completed it may be that, whatever values are used, the decision arrived at is always the same. If this is the case, the matter is closed. If, however, the choice is influenced by the particular values, among the plausible ones, that are used in the analysis, then either it really makes little difference whether or not testing is done because the benefits and costs are nearly equal, or there is a difference between benefit and costs, but the information available with which to discover it is not sufficiently precise. Since it is possible to determine for which items the imprecision is causing particular difficulty in arriving at a choice, it is possible to assign priorities to new research relevant to the question. The research dealing with more clearly determining costs of tests, illness, and death [item (d) above] is the domain of a different book. But in many instances the main item for which there is uncertainty is item (c), the degree of improvement in outcome associated with the patient being tested. The means available for reducing this uncertainty are the subject of the Chapter 3.

QUESTIONS, CHAPTER 2

2-1. Three hundred men hospitalized for symptoms of urinary obstruction were evaluated for cancer of the prostate gland. Among the tests performed by their physicians (board-certified urologists) was a digital rectal examination. The determination of an examination result as "positive" was made according to standard criteria, primarily, the presence of nodular irregularities or induration, and without knowledge of the results of other tests or of needle biopsy. The correspondence of the results of digital examination with those of biopsy is shown below (Guinan et al., 1980):

Biopsy positive for prostate cancer	Digital examination result: Positive	Negative	Total
Yes	48	21	69
No	25	206	231
Total	73	227	300

We will assume that the biopsy results are completely accurate in assessing the presence or absence of prostate cancer.

   a. In this population of men, what are the sensitivity and specificity of the digital examination for the presence of prostate cancer?
   b. In this population of men, what is the predictive value of a positive result of a digital examination? A negative result?
   c. You are a primary care physician considering administering an annual digital rectal examination to every male in your practice who is over 50 years of age, regardless of symptoms. From reviewing the literature, you suspect the prevalence of prostate cancer in this group to be about 0.5%. (i) Using the sensitivity and specificity obtained in 2.1a for the men with urological symptoms, calculate the fraction of men with a positive digital examination result who should prove to have prostate cancer. (ii) This proportion (predictive value of a postitive test) is lower than the one calculated in 2.1b. Why? (iii) What reservations do you have in applying the values for sensitivity and specificity of the digital examination obtained for the urological patients to values that might be found in your practice?

2-2. A common cause of death in persons with coronary heart disease is ventricular fibrillation (VF). To some extent, VF can be predicted by the presence of ventricular premature beats (VPB) on the electrocardiogram (ECG), and, to some extent, it can be prevented by appropriate treatment.

The following data come from a hypothetical study comparing two methods of identifying VPB among men with coronary heart disease. In a sample of 924 men, 444 had no VPB on either a standard ECG (a recording of less than 1 minute) or during ambulatory ECG monitoring for a 24-hour period. The data below apply to the remainder of the men:

No. of VPB per hour during 24-hour monitoring	No. of patients	% of patients	
		≥1 VPB on standard ECG	0 VPB on standard ECG
1–9	247	4.9	95.1
10–49	120	33.3	66.7
≥50	113	69.9	30.1

From other data, you know that only men with 10 or more VPB per hour are at increased risk of VF. Your aim is to determine how adequately the results obtained from the more convenient, less expensive, standard ECG can reproduce those obtained during 24-hour monitoring.

a. What is the sensitivity of the standard ECG in detecting men with ≥10 VPB per hour?

b. What is the specificity of the standard ECG in detecting men with <10 VPB per hour?

c. What fraction of men with coronary heart disease with ≥1 VPB on the standard ECG have ≥10 VPB per hour?

d. What fraction of men with coronary heart disease with 0 VPB on the standard ECG have <10 VPB per hour?

e. The decision to employ the standard or the 24-hour ECG in these patients is a difficult one. Construct decision trees for the two options (option 1: standard ECG followed by 24-hour ECG for persons with one or more VPB; option 2: 24-hour ECG for all patients) that highlight the key issues in the decision (Assume that VF is uniformly fatal.)

f. For which components of the trees are data available from the above study?

g. You estimate the relevant costs as follows: standard ECG, $35; 24-hour ECG, $200; antiarrhythmic therapy and monitoring for 1 year, $1,500; loss of life, $100,000. Assume that the probability of death from VF in the next year (at which time there would be a reevaluation for arrhythmic activity in all patients) is (i) 5.9% in persons with no or <10 VPB per hour; (ii) 11.5% in untreated persons with ≥10 VPB per hour; and (iii) 10.0% in persons with ≥10 VPB per hour who are given antiarrhythmic therapy. Which of the two options for screening for VPB is more cost-effective? If antiarrhythmic therapy reduced VF mortality to 8.0%, would your answer be the same?

h. Consider a third option in dealing with the problem of VF: no screening for VPB. Under the above assumptions, how does this policy compare with the other two?

ANSWERS

2-1.a. Sensitivity = 48/69 = 69.6%
Specificity = 206/231 = 89.2%

b. PV+ = 48/73 = 65.8%
PV− = 206/227 = 90.7%

c(i). In a population of 10,000 men in which 50 have prostate cancer:

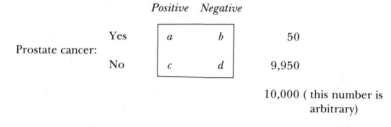

Digital examination:

		Positive	Negative	
	Yes	a	b	50
Prostate cancer:				
	No	c	d	9,950

10,000 (this number is arbitrary)

a = 50 (48/69) = 35
b = 50 − a = 15
d = 9,950 (206/231) = 8,873
c = 9950 − d = 1,077

Digital examination:

		Positive	Negative	
	Yes	35	15	50
Prostate cancer:				
	No	1,077	8,873	9,950
		1,112	8,888	10,000

PV+ = 35/1,112 × 100 = 3.1%

c(ii). Only 3.1% of your screened patients who have a positive digital exam will turn out to have prostate cancer. This PV+ is lower than that obtained for the men with urological symptoms because the prevalence of prostate cancer differs so much between the groups: 0.5% in the asymptomatic men versus 23% (69/300) in those with urological symptoms.

c(iii). Since most of the patients that you are examining will not have urological symptoms, the average size of any tumors that are present will probably be smaller than that found in a series of symptomatic men. Thus, the ability of the digital examination to detect true-positives in this group may be lower (i.e., lower sensitivity). Also, the sensitivity of the examination may be related to the skill of the person performing it; quite possibly the urologists are more adept at this examination than you. These two factors, which could act to decrease the sensitivity of digital examination in your patients relative to that found in the published study, would also somewhat lower the PV+.

   The specificity of the digital examination obtained in the study also may not predict that which you would achieve in your practice. Again, your relative lack of
expertise may lead to a relatively greater proportion of false-positives (i.e., lower
specificity). On the other hand, unlike in the published study, among your screened
patients who do not have prostate cancer the large majority will not have other
prostate abnormalities that could mimic cancer on the digital examination. Thus,
your proportion of false-positives could actually be smaller, leading to a higher
PV+ than that estimated in c(i) above.
   The moral of the story: Results of diagnostic tests performed by others, on
patient populations other than the one you are dealing with, can only be a *guide* to
how well the test will perform for you. How good a guide they will be is a function
of the variability of the test when performed by different individuals (laboratories,
radiology departments, etc.) as well as the similarity of the populations being tested.

2-2.

		Standard ECG:		
		≥1 VPB	0 VPB	Total
24-hour ECG:	≥10	119	114	233
	<10	12	679	691
(VPB/hour)	Total	131	793	924

a.   Sensitivity = 119/233 = 0.511

b.   Specificity = 679/691 = 0.983

c.   PV+ = 119/131 = 0.908

d.   PV− = 679/793 = 0.856

e,f.

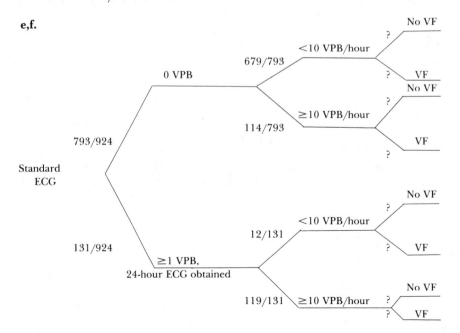

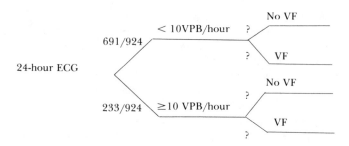

g,h. Death from VF in patients with coronary heart disease exacts a heavy toll on society. The average "cost" per patient per year exceeds $7,000, no matter which of the policies is adopted:

| | Cost (per year) when mortality in treated patients equals: | |
Policy	10%	8%
1. Standard ECG, with 24-hour ECG for "positives"	$7,376.75	$7,118.30
2. 24-hour ECG for all	$7,508.00	$7,004.00
3. No ECG	$7,311.20	$7,311.20

A reduction in mortality from VF in treated patients to only 10% (from 11.5%) is not enough to offset the costs of identifying patients with VPB (by either method) and treating them. On the other hand, once VF mortality in treated patients falls to 8%, it is most cost-effective to identify as many of the patients with ≥ 10 VPB per hour as possible, that is, to adopt a policy of 24-hour ECG monitoring for all such patients. At present, it is not known which figure more accurately reflects the mortality reduction. Both figures are plausible, and studies to determine which one is more plausible are needed to resolve the question.

REFERENCES

Bell RS, Loop JW: The utility and futility of radiographic skull examination for trauma. *N Engl J Med* 1971; 284:236–239.

Galen RS, Gambino SR: *Beyond Normality: The Predictive Value and Efficiency of Medical Diagnoses.* New York, John Wiley, 1975.

Guinan P, Bush I, Ray V, et al. The accuracy of the rectal examination in the diagnosis of prostate carcinoma. *N Engl. J Med* 1980; 303:499–503.

Royal College of Radiologists: Costs and benefits of skull radiography for head injury. *Lancet* 1981; 2:791–795.

3 Diagnostic and Screening Tests: Measuring Their Role in Improving the Outcome of Illness

To a large extent, the decision to perform or not perform a test depends on the degree to which the recognition of those persons who test positively can reduce the likelihood of disease occurring or progressing, or of complications developing. In the example described in previous chapters, the decision to use the Hemoccult test would be favored to the extent that mortality from colorectal cancer was reduced in a screened vis-à-vis an unscreened group. The decision to obtain a skull x-ray routinely in patients with head trauma, rather than select patients for x-ray examination on the basis of clinical criteria, is favored to the extent that adverse neurologic outcomes and death are associated with *not* identifying a skull fracture soon after injury.

Ordering or performing a diagnostic or screening test can reduce the frequency of disease occurrence/progression/complications only if the test can (a) detect the condition or abnormality before it or its consequences would otherwise be evident, and (b) lead to effective treatment. For a screening test, the treatment that follows the identification of the condition must be more effective when administered soon after the time of testing than when administered later in the natural history of the condition.

For most tests, information as to whether each of these requirements is met is generated in separate studies. Thus, the British study described in Chapter 2 evaluated the ability of clinical criteria and skull roentogenography to predict the occurrence of intracranial hematoma [requirement (a) above]. A study of a very different type, perhaps one that compared mortality in treated and untreated patients having intracranial hematoma diagnosed by skull roentgenography, would be needed to determine if the therapy available was efficacious [requirement (b) above].

A single study that attempts to determine if both requirements are met is usually far less feasible than either of the two component investigations. For example, consider the design of a single study that seeks to determine if there is any difference in mortality resulting from a policy of ordering skull x-ray films for all patients with head trauma and a policy of ordering skull x-ray films only for patients who test "positive" according to the clinical criteria. In the course of the study it would be necessary to (a) identify patients with head trauma treated according to each policy, (b) monitor mortality in both groups, and (c) assemble patient groups large enough to assure a meaningful comparison of death rates in clinically "negative" patients. Since in the British study in Chapter 2 there were no deaths (and only one intracranial hematoma) in the sample of 3,328 clinically negative patients who underwent skull roentgenography, it would be necessary to have two groups, each with considerably more patients than in this sample. An undertaking of such magnitude is to be avoided if at all possible!

Whether formally or informally, the overwhelming majority of commonly employed tests have been evaluated by the "two-step" process. For example, coronary arteriography has been evaluated for its ability to identify occlusive lesions and its own acute morbidity and mortality (step 1). The effect of bypass surgery for occlusive lesions found by anteriography on reducing subsequent mortality and on improving functional capacity has been studied separately (Principal Investigators of CASS and Associates, 1983a,b) (step 2). By combining the results of this sequence of studies with the monetary costs involved (see Chapter 1), it is possible to make an informed recommendation regarding coronary arteriography to a patient with angina pectoris. Similarly, various tests, from microscopic examination of red blood cells to analyses of certain serum constituents, have been evaluated for their abilities to determine the presence and type of anemia (step 1). Once the efficacy of treatment of the types of anemia is determined (step 2), it is possible to estimate the the degree to which testing for the presence and type of anemia will lead to reduced morbidity from these conditions.

Methods for quantifying the adequacy with which a test measures what it intends to was the subject of Chapter 2. Methods for quantifying the extent to which treatment is efficacious are discussed in Chapters 4 and 5, but suffice it to say here that such methods generally require two groups of patients with a positive test or a specific condition, one treated and the other untreated (or treated in another manner). But what is to be done if all patients who are found to be "positive" on a certain test happen to receive treatment? Persons who are tested for cancer and found to have it, for example, are almost never left untreated. Thus, while it is not difficult to determine that a number of screening tests for cancer can detect the disease earlier than it would be detected otherwise (e.g., by comparing the distribution of tumor size or stage in tested and untested persons with that cancer), it is usually not possible to answer the second necessary question—does treatment given at the time of early detection lead to a more favorable outcome than treatment given when the cancer is clinically manifest? In situations such as this, it is necessary to resort to the one-step, often exceedingly cumbersome, design referred to earlier, that is, the comparison of the subsequent occurrence of progression/complications in tested and untested persons. This chapter outlines the types of one-step studies available to measure the efficacy of a test.

EXPERIMENTAL AND NONEXPERIMENTAL FOLLOW-UP STUDIES

The groups to be compared, tested versus not tested, can be defined by the investigator, with subjects assigned at random to one group or the other. Alternatively, it is possible to exploit (with appropriate caution) the fact that in the normal course of medical/public health practice some persons are tested while others are not, and these two groups can be monitored for the outcome(s) of interest.

An example of the first type, an *experimental* evaluation, is the study conducted at the Kaiser Health Plan on the efficacy of multiphasic screening (Cutler et al., 1973). Beginning in 1964, some 5,000 members of the Plan born during the years 1910 to 1929 were invited to undergo an annual examination that had a number of components: history, physical examination, selected blood and urine tests, chest and breast roentgenography, sigmoidoscopy, and measurement of vision, hearing, and respiratory function. The subjects were selected from a group of more than 40,000 members who were potentially eligible on the basis of the terminal digit of their sequentially assigned medical record numbers. A group of similar size with a different terminal digit was identified for purposes of comparison, and these members did not receive the invitation. In the years that followed, the two groups were compared regarding the frequency of outpatient visits and hospitalizations, disability (ascertained by a mail questionnaire), and mortality.

The second approach to measuring the value of testing, *nonexperimental follow-up* evaluation, is exemplified by the comparison of neonatal mortality among children delivered by mothers who received fetal monitoring during labor with that among children whose mothers had not been monitored (Neutra et al., 1978). The study took place in a U.S. hospital during the late 1960s to early 1970s, a period in which fetal monitoring was being introduced there. The decision as to which women were to undergo monitoring was made by the individual physicians, not by the investigators (who, indeed, conducted the study in retrospect through the use of the hospital's records).

Ideally, all evaluations of diagnostic or screening test efficacy would be experimental: Assignment of patients to test or no-test groups in a random way assures that the only differences between the two groups that might be relevant to the outcome in question are those that occur by chance. This is decidedly not the case in nonexperimental studies, as all too often there are important differences that have the potential to distort (confound) the true benefit, or lack thereof, associated with the test. In the fetal monitoring study, for example, the investigators discovered in their review of records that the mothers who did not receive monitoring had characteristics more often than did the monitored mothers that predict an increased risk of mortality in the child: short gestation, breech presentation, placenta previa, and so on. Failure to have taken into account these differences in the analysis would have resulted in a comparison erroneously favorable to the monitored group and would have led to an overestimation of the benefit associated with monitoring.

Unfortunately, even when it is possible in the course of a nonexperimental study to measure and to take into account (see Chapter 8) the influence of some confounding variables, it is never possible to be sure that there are not others. It is impossible to say, for example, that there were not reasons other than, for example, short gestation or breech presentation for administering fetal monitoring to women that also had a strong bearing on neonatal mortality. The likelihood with which unmeasured factors are biasing (confounding) the results can be guessed at, as can the degree to which they may be doing so. Nonetheless, while the results of nonexperimental studies are often used in arriving at decisions regarding the use of diagnostic and screening tests, they are never as "satisfying" as would be the same results from an otherwise comparable experimental study. (Also see Chapter 5 for a more complete discussion of the strengths and limitations of nonexperimental evaluations.)

There are some nonexperimental follow-up studies in which the potential for this sort of bias is particularly clear. Perhaps you are attempting to evaluate the success of a blood lead screening program for preschool children in which the test was available to all who requested it. The program's "success" would be measured by IQ testing of these children once they were of school age, and their performance would be compared with that of an unscreened group. Without having been able to assign children to the test or no-test categories, you are fearful that the two groups of children may have IQ differences based on a number of other factors (e.g., parental IQ differences) apart from any benefit the screening program may have had. It may even be that the screened children had some neurological or behavioral problems that were the reason for their being tested. Without being able to identify these other factors and measure them comparably in screened and unscreened children, the results of any comparison will have little credibility.

Nonexperimental evaluations of the efficacy of screening for cancer provide another example of the problems involved in interpreting results when the action of confounding factors is suspected. To this day, some uncertainty remains regarding the efficacy of the Pap smear in reducing mortality from cervical cancer, partly due to the fact that experimental studies have not been conducted and partly because nonexperimental comparisons of screened and unscreened women could easily be biased by the fact that the two groups are known or suspected to be at very different risks of developing invasive cervical cancer.

While confounding can occur in experimental studies of test efficacy as well, it is not usually as great a concern. It only occurs when the subjects assigned to the test and no-test groups have, by chance, different probabilities of disease progression/complications. (Randomization will produce equality of groups on the average, although in an individual study there can be differences). Nonetheless, if there are some characteristics that are known to relate strongly to the likelihood of progression/complications, it is advisable not to rely solely on randomization to prevent confounding. For example, a study conducted at the Health Insurance Plan of New York randomly assigned women to groups in which they were

either offered annual screening for breast cancer or no intervention, in an effort to determine if early detection could influence
mortality rates from this disease (Shapiro et al., 1971). However, the
randomization was performed in such a way as to guarantee that the
two groups were identical with respect to age and family size, since
these were readily identified characteristics that are associated with
breast cancer mortality.

WHICH SUBJECTS ARE TO BE COMPARED?

In most evaluations of the efficacy of diagnostic or screening tests,
the only comparison that can be made is of the overall occurrence
of progression/complications in the screened versus unscreened
groups. In a blood lead screening evaluation, for instance, one
would compare the prevalence of retardation in children who did
and did not receive screening. The lead levels in the unscreened
group would never be known, and so even if the investigators
wished to compare outcomes in only those persons with elevated
levels in each group, it would be impossible to do so.

However, some conditions for which testing is done will, after a
period of time, be evident even without benefit of the test. Most
cancers fall into this category, and there has been a temptation to
evaluate the efficacy of cancer screening tests by comparing mortality from the particular cancer in cases found through screening
with that in other cases. Giving in to this temptation will lead to
erroneous results, primarily due to the influence of what is known
as lead-time bias.

The reason for this bias is illustrated in the following example.
Suppose 100 individuals are screened for cancer X, a cancer for
which there is no effective treatment. On the average, the test suc-
ceeds in identifying the cancer 1 year before it is clinically evident.
Four persons in the group are detected as having cancer X, and the
course of their illness is shown in Fig. 3-1.

Two deaths occur among the four persons with cancer X in the
13 person-years that occur following screening $(3 + 4 + 2 + 4$,
see Figure 3-1), and their mortality rate is 2 per 13 person-years.
Had the screening *not* been performed, however, the same two
deaths among 4 cases in 100 persons would occur (since no effective
treatment follows early detection). But the number of person-years
accruing in these cases from the time of their diagnosis (1 year later

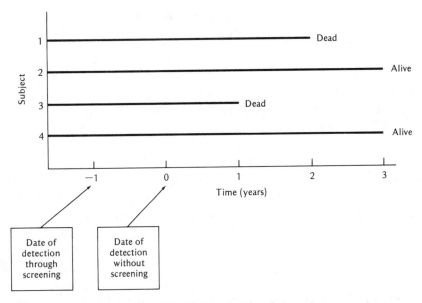

Figure 3-1. Lead time in studies of the efficacy of screening.

than that for the screened cases) would be only 9 (2 + 3 + 1 + 3) and the resulting mortality rate would be higher, 2 per 9 person-years. Since screening could not lead to improved mortality, one must conclude that there is something faulty in this method of comparison. (If, instead of using mortality rates, the measure of outcome were n-year survival, the bias would still be present. Thus, the 1.5-year survival in the cases found through screening is 100%, whereas the 1.5-year survival in the other cases is 75%, even though the two groups had, in truth, an identical survival experience.)

What is faulty, of course, is that the starting point for monitoring mortality rates is different between the screened and unscreened cases, always to the apparent detriment of the cases detected without screening. The appropriate comparison to make is the mortality experience (with respect to that cancer), not of the cases alone but of the screened group with that of an unscreened group, *with both groups monitored from the time of screening.* In the above example, the mortality rate in the screened group is 2 deaths in 397 person-years (98 persons × 4 years, plus 1 person × 2 years, plus 1 person × 3 years). In a comparable unscreened group, the rate would be the same since the number of person-years, counted from the time the screening would have taken place had it been done, is identical to that for the screened group. Given that the natural history of this cancer is not altered by screening, this comparison, which indicates no benefit associated with screening, is clearly the preferred one.[1]

OTHER APPROACHES TO MEASURING THE DEGREE TO WHICH TESTS REDUCE THE OCCURRENCE OF PROGRESSION/COMPLICATIONS

Population Comparisons

Let's say you are interested in determining if the routine use of skull roentgenography in patients with head trauma reduces trauma-associated mortality in comparison with a policy of obtaining x-ray films only in patients who are clinically positive. You despair of obtaining the resources necessary to identify and follow the large number of persons needed for a nonexperimental follow-up study, and a randomized trial seems even less feasible. What about simply comparing the mortality rates from traumatic intracranial hematoma in two or more populations whose experience differs regarding the routine use of skull x-ray films? The "populations" could be defined, for example, according to residence in certain geographic areas or to the hospital emergency room in which care was provided. Data would have to be available on the frequency of the complication (e.g., death from intracranial hematoma) and, at least roughly, on the degree to which one or the other of the testing strategies (i.e., clinical criteria vs. routine skull roentgenography) had been employed in the respective populations. What is not needed for this type of comparison is the more difficult to come by knowledge of both test and complication status in individual patients—if these were known, a nonexperimental follow-up design could be used.

While population comparisons offer a relatively inexpensive and rapid means of assessing test efficacy, it is only under unusual circumstances that the evidence they provide can be considered any-

---

[1]Patients who have a long preclinical-but-detectable phase of disease are more readily found via screening than are patients whose preclinical phase is short. To the extent that the length of the preclinical phase correlates with the length of the illness once it has been detected, those persons whose disease was found via screening will appear to have a better survival rate, even in the absence of treatment that influences the disease's natural history. This artifact, due to what has been termed "length-biased sampling" (Zelen, 1976), is another reason that a comparison of survival in persons whose disease was detected by screening with that of other diseased persons will be misleading.

thing more than suggestive. This is because, unfortunately, it is uncommon to find populations which differ to a large degree in the use they make of a diagnostic or screening test but which are otherwise similar with respect to (a) the rate of occurrence of the outcome that can result from progression/complications of the condition for which testing is being done, and (b) the completeness and accuracy of the reporting of this outcome.

Occurrence of the Condition

One way to evaluate the efficacy of a blood lead screening program in reducing the prevalence of mental retardation is to compare the prevalence of the retardation in the screened population with that of one or more unscreened populations. The latter would be chosen on the basis of characteristics that would predict a frequency of retardation identical to that of the screened population, save for the influence of screening. Such characteristics might be geographic proximity to the screened population, income level, age and type of housing, and the use of similar methods of identifying retarded children.

The difficulty in interpreting the results of such a comparison is that we are never very sure that, despite our best efforts in selecting control communities, the "background" prevalences of retardation among the populations were indeed similar. Might the difference (or lack thereof) we observe in the prevalence of retardation have been present in the absence of screening? This is particularly a problem if the screening measure, by its nature, is unlikely to have a dramatic impact on the overall occurrence of the complication or condition it seeks to prevent. For instance, because lead exposure may be responsible for only a relatively small fraction of the retardation that occurs among children, even an effective screening program may make only a small dent in the overall prevalence, which would be hard to detect against the background level.

Completeness and Accuracy of Reporting

Often it is difficult to obtain any reliable population data on the occurrence of the progression/complication of interest, particularly in a population group large enough to provide enough instances of progression/complications for a meaningful comparison. For example, even if two hospitals with different policies regarding skull roentgenography had similar criteria for determining the presence of intracranial hematoma and had records that allowed the occurrence of this complication to be determined, it is unlikely that there would be sufficient patients with head trauma to generate enough intracranial hematoma cases to permit the comparison of mortality rates between them. Yet, data on the occurrence of intracranial hematoma in a larger population, such as a city, county, or state, can rarely be obtained, and so the case-fatality comparisons between these populations cannot be made.

Occasionally, the circumstances under which population comparisons are made allow results to be interpreted with relatively great confidence.

> *Example.* A program of cervical screening of Icelandic women aged 25 to 59 years was begun in 1964. Whereas only occasionally would a woman have received screening prior to that time, by the early 1970s some 80% of the target population had been examined at the screening clinic. Some women 60 years and over attended the clinic as well, but not in any appreciable numbers until after 1970. The mortality from cervical cancer and the incidence of lesions of Stage II or greater are shown in Table 3-1. In 25- to 59-year-old women, a rise both in mortality and the incidence of late-stage disease during 1955–69 was reversed in 1970–74. In the women 60 to 89 years old, the group that underwent little screening, there was no systematic variation in either rate during the interval (Johannesson, 1978).

Was it the screening that was responsible for this difference between the "populations" (i.e., the 25- to 59-year-old Icelandic women before and after the mass screening)? Features of the study's design and results that favor an affirmative answer to this question are as follows:

1. The difference in the level of screening between the time periods was very great, rising from near zero before 1964 to 80% within 10 years.

Table 3-1. Cervical Cancer in Iceland, 1955 to 1974

Age (years)	Measure	Rate of cervical cancer[a]			
		1955–59	1960–64	1965–69	1970–74
25–59	Mortality	11.7	16.8	26.5	12.2
	Incidence, Stage II+	16.8	19.3	22.3	11.8
60–89	Mortality	27.6	33.3	28.2	34.8
	Incidence, Stage II+	27.8	21.0	25.4	23.1

[a]Annual rate per 100,000, age-adjusted (5-year groups) to a uniform standard.
Source: Johannesson et al. (1978).

2. Reliable data were available on the mortality from cervical cancer.
3. The size of the population in each time period was sufficiently large to provide enough cervical cancer deaths for meaningful analysis.
4. There is evidence to indicate that, in the absence of screening, the mortality rates among 25- to 59-year-old women would not have fallen: (a) prior to the introduction of mass screening, the rates in women in this age group actually had been on the increase, and (b) in those Icelandic women who were largely unscreened, that is, women aged 60 to 89, there was no corresponding decrease in mortality from cervical cancer during 1970 to 1974.
5. The mortality (and late-stage incidence) in 1970 to 1974 was reduced to such a large degree that it is implausible that other, unmeasured changes during the period could have been solely responsible.

These are precisely the features that are rarely present *together* in most comparisons of populations.

Case-Control Studies

The case-control approach is particularly valuable when studying disease etiology and plays an important role in evaluating therapeutic safety (see Chapter 6). It examines potential associations between exposures and disease in an apparently illogical way, by comparing the frequency (or level) of exposure in a group of persons having disease with that in an otherwise comparable group of persons without it. While the opportunity for bias in such studies is considerable (as is the case for any nonexperimental study), if properly done they can provide an accurate estimate of the relative disease incidence in exposed and nonexposed persons (Cornfield, 1951) and can do so in an efficient way.

How can this type of study design be put to use to evaluate the efficacy of a diagnostic or screening test? "Cases" would have to be defined as individuals who have developed progressive disease or complications that one is seeking to prevent by prompt diagnosis. "Controls" would be defined as persons without progression/complications but who are otherwise comparable. Thus, if the cases were persons who died of intracranial hematoma following head trauma despite having been clinically negative, the controls would be persons with head trauma of equal severity, also clinically negative, who did not die. Records of the two groups would be examined to determine in which patients an x-ray film of the skull had been obtained at the time of first presentation. The data would be displayed as follows:

Death from intracranial hematoma:

		Yes	No
Skull x-ray test:	Performed	a	b
	Not performed	c	d

In clinically negative persons, routine skull x-ray films would be effective in reducing mortality in proportion to the amount by which $b/(b + d)$ exceeded $a/(a + c)$.

The use of the case-control study to measure the efficacy of diagnostic tests has, to the present time, been more a theoretical possibility than a reality. This is the result of the fact that the conditions required for such studies—a large patient population for which data regarding symptoms are uniformly available and within which there is variation in the way in which (or speed with which) diagnostic tests are used—have rarely been present.

Case-control studies of the efficacy of screening tests have proven somewhat more feasible primarily because there is often more variability in the fact or frequency of screening in healthy persons than in the use of diagnostic tests in sick ones. Three features of the design and analysis of case-control studies of screening efficacy are worthy of mention:

1. Persons selected as cases should be ill or disabled to a degree that diagnosis would occur in the absence of screening (Morrison, 1982). For a disease such as cancer, the criterion for selection could be death from cancer and/or the presence of symptomatic and extensive illness, irrespective of the stage at which the cancer was first diagnosed. In choosing cases for a study of blood lead screening and mental retardation, particular care would have to be taken to set criteria stringent enough so that, in the study locale, cases of defined severity would be reliably identified even if no screening program existed.

2. Persons selected as controls should be representative of the

population that generated the cases with respect to the presence and/or level of screening activity (Weiss, 1983). To the extent that they can be identified, persons with earlier or less severe forms of the condition under study (e.g., low-stage cancer) will rarely be suitable for this purpose. The fact that the condition is detected early in such persons is probably the result of their frequently seeking or performing screening. Thus, even if screening were not followed by any effective therapy, a case-control difference would exist, one that would falsely claim a benefit associated with screening. A bias of this sort is the case-control analogue of lead-time bias in follow-up studies (see p. 38). While the appropriate control group would not exclude persons with early or mild disease, it would include them only in proportion to their numbers in the population. (What specifically constitutes an "appropriate" control group in a case-control study is a question that is discussed more fully in Chapter 6.)

Thus, in a case-control study that seeks to determine if cytologic screening for cervical cancer leads to a reduction in the mortality from the disease, one would not choose as controls women with in situ lesions. The presence of in situ cervical neoplasia is rarely discovered in the absence of screening, and so virtually every member of the control group will have had at least one examination. It is unlikely that such a high level of screening activity would occur among women in the population that gave rise to the patients who died from cervical cancer. The selection of women with in situ cancer as controls would produce a finding of apparent benefit from cytologic screening even if there were no effective treatment for the lesions discovered in this way.

Example. To date, several case-control studies have been conducted to estimate the degree to which mortality from breast cancer might be reduced by early detection through regular breast self-examination (BSE). The designs of the studies were similar: Women whose cancers were diagnosed at late and early stages (i.e., cases and controls, respectively) were compared with respect to the frequency of BSE. This design violates both principles thus far enumerated:

(a) The goal of early detection is to prevent the occurrence of late-stage disease at any time, not merely at diagnosis. Thus, the criteria for selection of "cases" should not have been based solely on information available at the time of diagnosis. The impact on the results when cases are chosen in this manner is uncertain. Since some late-stage cases are asymptomatic, some will have been detected by BSE, and this will lead to a low estimate of BSE efficacy. On the other hand, many of the cases which should have but did not appear in these studies, that is, women who developed late-stage breast cancer at some time after the initial diagnosis of their disease, once had early cancer found by BSE. Their exclusion could falsely inflate the measured efficacy of BSE.

(b) The BSE practices of women with breast cancer diagnoses at an early stage are almost certainly not typical of those of the population of women from which the late-stage cases arose. In most instances, BSE or other early detection activity will have been responsible for the early diagnosis. Restriction of the control group to these women with higher-than-average early detection activity will cause the control-case difference in the frequency of BSE to be falsely large.

3. As is the case with all nonexperimental strategies for assessing the efficacy of screening, there is a possibility of obtaining a spurious result unless factors that are correlated both with the level of screening activity and the occurrence of late-stage disease/mortality are taken into account. Factors can be related to the occurrence of late-stage disease by virtue of their relationship to disease incidence per se or to the likelihood of disease progression or spread. Thus, in a study of BSE and late breast cancer it would be necessary to evaluate (and possibly adjust for) characteristics that are associated with breast cancer incidence (e.g., race and educational level) and that differ between cases and controls. Similarly, adjustment would have to be made if women who regularly performed BSE also more commonly received the benefit of other detection methods for breast cancer (e.g., mammography and clinical examination), if the analysis found these other methods to have been efficacious.

QUESTION, CHAPTER 3

3-1. The 5-year survival of men with localized cancer of the prostate gland is about 60%, whereas that for men with regional involvement from this disease is about 50%. A new test has been developed that, if applied in asymptomatic men, will enable all cases to be diagnosed at the localized stage. The test is inexpensive and innocuous. The developers of the test claim that if the test is used in asymptomatic men, mortality rates from prostate cancer will decrease. What reservations do you have regarding this claim?

ANSWER

3-1. It is not necessarily true that mortality rates from carcinoma of the prostate will diminish following implementation of the new test. From the data presented, we do not even know if it is more advantageous to diagnose a case of prostate cancer at the localized stage than at the regional stage. The difference in 5-year survival between the two groups, 60% versus 50%, could conceivably be due to lead-time bias. Second, we are unable to tell from these data whether the cases previously diagnosed at the regional stage would have had a better prognosis if they had been diagnosed at the localized stage. It may be that these are men with inherently more aggressive tumors, which, irrespective of stage of diagnosis, would produce high mortality.

What is required to evaluate the efficacy of the new test in reducing mortality rates from prostate cancer is either one of the following two approaches: (a) a one-step study, in which groups of men who do and do not receive the test are monitored for mortality rate from prostate cancer from the time of testing; or (b) the second step of a two-step study (we already have the results of the first step, which showed the test to be capable of detecting localized disease) in which men diagnosed as having cancer of the prostate by this new test are randomly allocated to treatment or no-treatment groups. This second approach is a theoretical possibility only, since it is not considered ethical at the present time.

REFERENCES

Cornfield J: A method of estimating comparative rates from clinical data. Application to cancer of the lung, breast, and cervix. *JNCI* 1951; 11:1269-1275.

Cutler JL, Ramcharan S, Feldman R, et al.: Multiphasic checkup evaluation study. 1. Methods and population. *Prev Med* 1973; 2:197-206.

Johannesson G, Geirsson G, Day N: The effect of mass screening in Iceland, 1965–74, on the incidence and mortality of cervical carcinoma. *Int J Cancer* 1978; 21:418-425.

Morrison AS: Case definition in case-control studies of the efficacy of screening. *Am J Epidemiol* 1982; 115:6-8.

Neutra RR, Fienberg SE, Greenland S, et al.: Effect of fetal monitoring on neonatal death rates. *N Engl J Med* 1978; 299:324-326.

Principal Investigators of CASS and Associates (Killip T, ed, and Fisher LD, Mock MB, assoc eds): Coronary artery surgery study: A randomized trial of coronary artery bypass surgery—Survival data. *Circulation* 1983a; 68:939-950.

Principal Investigators of CASS and Associates (Killip T, ed, and Fisher LD, Mock MB, assoc eds): Coronary artery surgery study: A randomized trial of coronary artery bypass surgery—Quality of life in patients randomly assigned to treatment groups. *Circulation* 1983b; 68:951-960.

Shapiro S, Strax P, Venet L: Periodic breast cancer screening in reducing mortality from breast cancer. *JAMA* 1971; 215:1777-1785.

Weiss NS: Control definition in case-control studies of the efficacy of screening and diagnostic testing. *Am J Epidemiol* 1983; 118:457-460.

Zelen M: Theory of early detection of breast cancer in the general population, in Hensen JC, Mattheim WH, Rozencweig M (eds): *Breast Cancer: Trends in Research and Treatment.* New York, Raven Press, 1976.

4 Therapeutic Efficacy: Experimental Studies

An experimental study of therapeutic efficacy is one in which (a) patients are assigned to one of two or more groups to be offered different therapeutic measures, (b) chance alone dictates whether a particular patient will be assigned to a particular group, and (c) patients in each group are monitored for the abatement of their illness or for the occurrence of the event(s) that the therapy seeks to prevent. Commonly used synonyms for this type of study are "clinical trial" and "randomized controlled trial."

Experimental designs provide results that can be interpreted relatively easily, for the common concern in nonexperimental studies—that the various treatment groups had inherently unequal probabilities of doing well—is much less pressing when it is only chance that determines the membership of the groups. For this reason, the popularity of experimental studies has increased during the last several decades. The approach has been applied to virtually every class of therapy, from pharmaceutical agents to surgical techniques to dietary and other "life-style" interventions.

The concept of an experimental study is straightforward. However, a number of issues that are not so straightforward have to be considered when planning the design and analysis of a particular study. The ways in which these issues are dealt with often have a substantial bearing on the validity and interpretation of the results.

CHOOSING THE SUBJECTS FOR STUDY

Generalizing Beyond the Study Population

The rationale for research in clinical epidemiology (and in all other health research in humans) is that by observing the illness experience of some persons we may come away with lessons that can be applied elsewhere. So, by determining that persons randomly assigned to receive drug A fare better than those assigned to receive drug B, we can conclude that persons similar to those in the study will do better on the average by taking drug A rather than drug B.

To what extent must these two groups—study subjects and persons to whom we would like to refer the findings (reference population)—be "similar" so that valid generalizations can be made from one to the other? To answer this question, it is necessary to take into account the answers to two other questions: (a) Do both the study and reference populations suffer untoward consequences from the condition for which the therapy is being given? (b) If the therapy is effective in the study population, would the means by which it is believed to act (i.e., its biological effect) be present in members of the reference population as well?

To illustrate how the matter of generalizing is approached in practice, let's place ourselves back in the late 1960s, immediately following the publication of the results of the first, large, randomized controlled trial of antihypertensive therapy for the reduction of mortality from cardiovascular disease (Veterans Administration Cooperative Study Group on Antihypertensive Agents, 1967). The study documented a substantial mortality reduction in actively treated versus placebo-treated male veterans with a diastolic blood pressure of 115 to 129 mm Hg who were free of clinical cardiac or cerebrovascular disease and in whom there was no advanced retinal or renal pathology. Now, let's say we had a patient with that level of blood pressure but who was neither a veteran nor male. Should we presume that the findings apply to her? Is an experimental study of the efficacy of antihypertensive drugs needed in non–war veteran women? We would address the issue by considering, first, whether high blood pressure in nonveterans and women predisposes them to an increased risk of mortality from cardiovascular diseases. In 1967, data were available indicating that such persons indeed were at increased risk. [Of course, there are other situations in which the available data suggest no relationship. For example, in hypertensive persons over the age of 75 years there may be little increased mortality over that in normotensive persons (Mitchell, 1983). Also, it may be that data just are not available for the population or disease subgroup to which a patient belongs that link the condition being treated with the outcome.]

Second, we would ask whether the postulated mechanism through which antihypertensive therapy exerted its beneficial effect on mortality in male veterans is present in nonveteran women. Unfortunately, it is rarely possible to arrive at an unequivocal answer to a question of this sort, for our knowledge of the pathogenetic mechanism(s) is rarely definitive. While there would be no basis for believing that nonveterans differ from veterans in this respect, it is not out of the question that hormonal and other differences between the sexes could make the extrapolation from men to women inexact. The uncertainty would almost certainly be greater still when trying to extrapolate the study results to persons with blood pressure levels below 115 mm Hg. The benefit of antihypertensive therapy would be expected to be smaller in them (for their excess risk is smaller), but by how much? This is no minor matter, as there is a far greater number of people with modest elevations of blood pressure than there is with large elevations, and at some point a blood pressure threshold must be set below which therapy will not be instituted.[1]

Maximizing the Study's Ability to Identify Therapeutic Efficacy

Some leap of faith is going to have to be made in applying the results obtained in the study subjects to the reference population. Therefore, the choice of the particular group of subjects for study usually depends less on the degree to which the group represents the reference population than on the group having characteristics that will produce a study with high "power," that is, characteristics that will successfully identify a difference between treatments, if one is truly present. There are two such important characteristics.

---

[1]By the end of the 1970s, experimental studies had demonstrated the efficacy of antihypertenisve therapy in nonveterans, women, and persons with less extreme blood pressure elevations. The Hypertension Detection and Follow-up Group (1979a,b) contrasted treatment by regular medical care with that by specialized centers that provided close blood pressure scrutiny and control. Persons randomly assigned to the specialized centers experienced a greater average reduction in blood pressure than did persons receiving regular care, and they had a lower mortality, irrespective of sex or initial diastolic blood pressure (≥90 mm Hg).

Low Cost of Enrolling and Monitoring Members of the Group

The lower the cost per subject, the larger will be the number of subjects available at a given budget level (it is necessary to get these studies funded!) and the more statistically powerful will be the study. An early investigation of the effect of a low–cholesterol, low–saturated fat diet on the incidence of cardiovascular disease was conducted in a Veterans Administration psychiatric hospital (Dayton et al., 1969). Patients receiving meals from one kitchen had a modified diet, whereas the diet of other patients remained as before. The cost of performing this intervention at an institution clearly was less than that of trying to modify dietary cholesterol and saturated fat on an individual basis in individual kitchens.

Once a group of investigators has been established to conduct a randomized controlled trial, there is an economy in having these same investigators conduct additional studies. The initial administrative costs can be avoided (and possibly also the costs that can be associated with the group's early inexperience) when another therapy for the disease first treated is to be evaluated, or when the investigators begin an evaluation of a therapy for another disease that they encounter. In some instances, the same patients enrolled and participating in the first study can be enrolled in the second study. For example, to determine if aspirin use could prevent myocardial reinfarction, participants in some treatment groups of the Coronary Drug Project that had been disbanded (e.g., those assigned to receive estrogen or thyroid hormones), but who were still under surveillance, were randomly assigned to receive aspirin or placebo (Coronary Drug Project Research Group, 1976).

High Expected Compliance with the Therapeutic Regimen(s) and Likelihood of Successful Follow-Up

Many clinical trials begin with a "run-in" phase in which all potential subjects are given a placebo or a "control" therapy. Their compliance with the regimen is assessed, and only those in whom compliance is good are entered into the randomized portion of the study (also see p. 58). This is yet another assault on the "representativeness" of the study subjects vis-à-vis the reference population, for the latter invariably would include volunteers and nonvolunteers, compliers and noncompliers, to whom one would like to extrapolate the results. Yet, the resulting study population offers a "clean" separation of subjects exposed to the various treatments, and thus enhances the ability to find any true between-treatment difference that might exist.

[Occasionally, a study has as its goal the measurement of efficacy in the population to whom the intervention is offered, that is, the efficacy in those who receive it combined with the dilution that results from whatever noncompliance exists in that population. For example, the study of mammography and clinical breast examination conducted within the Health Insurance Plan of New York randomly assigned some of the female members to the intervention group and only then notified them of the study (Shapiro et al., 1971). A sizable fraction of these women, 35%, failed to attend even a single screening examination. Nonetheless, since the aim of the study was to determine if screening of this type would reduce mortality from breast cancer in a population to whom it was offered, the aims of the study were served fully by comparing mortality in the study group, at whatever level of compliance, with that of other women in the Plan.]

NATURE OF THE INTERVENTION

Generalizing Beyond the Therapeutic Measure under Study

Often there are a number of interventions that can accomplish the same biochemical or physiologic change, for example, lowering serum cholesterol, lowering arterial blood pressure, raising gastric pH. If only one of the therapies has been evaluated (say, against a placebo) and a beneficial effect has been found in preventing or controlling a clinical manifestation that results from the original biochemical/physiological derangement, what can be said of the benefits expected from the use of another therapy that is believed to act in the same manner?

Here, just as with the question of generalizing from the study to the reference population, it is not possible to provide a definitive answer that covers all situations. To the extent that the means by which the evaluated therapy exerted its beneficial effect is (a) known and (b) shared by the not-yet-evaluated therapy, there will be confidence that it is also effective. Since this is a subjective assessment, not all who review the evidence will arrive at the same conclusion. For example, a decline in mortality from coronary disease was noted in persons assigned at random to take cholestyramine, an agent that lowers the concentration of certain serum lipids (Lipid Research

Clinics Program, 1984). Is it reasonable to assume that a diet that can accomplish a similar reduction in lipid levels will accomplish a similar reduction in mortality? Experts are not unanimous in their answers to this question, since they are not unanimous in believing that the effect of cholestyramine that is relevant to coronary disease is shared by a low–saturated fat, low-cholesterol diet.

Maximizing the Study's Ability to Identify Therapeutic Efficacy

The finding of no difference between treatments employed in a clinical trial often occurs because the true difference between the treatments is too small to have been reliably detected in the trial. At the planning stage of a clinical trial, there are two ways to try to make a false-negative result less likely: The number of subjects to be enrolled can be made large (see p. 51), or, the intervention chosen can be made as different as possible from that to be offered to the comparison group(s). For example, suppose you are evaluating the effect of dietary modification on disease (e.g., low saturated fat intake in relation to the occurrence of myocardial infarction, or, in older children with phenylketonuria, abridgement of low phenylalanine intake in relation to IQ). It would be important to make the modified diet as different as possible from that of the controls, within the range of what you believe will be acceptable to patients. There will always be critics of a "negative" study who say that, had the intervention only been somewhat more extreme, a positive result would have emerged. You want to avoid giving them any extra ammunition!

NATURE OF THE THERAPY TO BE ADMINISTERED TO THE COMPARISON GROUP

Typically, the comparison group is prescribed "conventional" therapy, which may range from no therapy at all to a complex array of interventions that is believed, at that time, to be the best that can be offered. To justify the conduct of the study, of course, there should be a "reasonable" probability that the comparison therapy, even if it is no therapy, will prove to be as good as or superior to the therapy under study. A judgment as to what is reasonable will be based on existing data, usually from nonexperimental studies. Since a judgment is involved, there often will be disagreement among investigators as to the adequacy of these data in determining the efficacy of the therapy being considered for study and thus there often will be disagreement as to whether it is ethical to subject some patients to any other therapy.

If some form of placebo is to be used it should be, if possible, totally innocuous. However, there are some situations in which the manipulation necessary to administer the therapy is such that, in the absence of a similar manipulation in the comparision group, the internal validity of the study could be undermined due to a placebo effect. One such situation arose in a clinical trial that evaluated the effect of an intradiskal injection of chymopapain to relieve sciatica due to a herniated lumbar disc (Javid et al., 1983). A needle was placed into the intervertebral disc of each study subject, who was then given either chymopapain or sterile saline on a random basis.

Since the administration of an intradiskal injection of an inert substance could never be considered a legitimate therapeutic alternative—it poses at least some risk and discomfort to the patient with no possibility of benefit—how can it be justified ethically? The only way is to have the prospective subjects informed as to the nature of the study and of the rationale for the use of a placebo that is not free of risk and/or discomfort. They can then decide whether they are willing to subject themselves to the risks so that others may benefit.

Experimental evaluations of coronary artery bypass surgery have eschewed the use of blinding by means of a "sham" surgical procedure, and have instead assigned comparison patients to "medical" therapy (Principal Investigators of CASS and Associates, 1981). When planning the studies the investigators believed that, in terms of some combination of pain relief, functional ability, and mortality, the medical therapy group might well have a better outcome than their surgical therapy counterparts. However, this choice of comparison therapy meant that certain important research questions could no longer be unambiguously addressed. Specifically, it would be impossible to determine if any reduced level of pain in the patients undergoing bypass surgery, relative to that in the medical therapy group, was a result of the bypass per se or simply of the more general effect of a surgical procedure performed within the chest (Cobb et al., 1959). Nonetheless, it would have been inappropriate to do anything other than place the patients' welfare first, even though that forced some of the goals of the studies to be compromised.

Clearly, this lack of blinding of subjects and investigators will prove more important in the interpretation of some outcomes (e.g., chest pain) than of others (e.g., mortality). If possible, of course, it is better to keep both subjects and investigators ignorant of the treatment status, as this will minimize the possibility of actions on the part of either group that could bias the results. When complications of disease or therapy arise that necessitate knowledge of the specific therapy to which the patient has been assigned, this information usually can be given to one or more physicians external to the study who can decide on the proper course of action. If the therapy under study is a drug, the blinding is generally done simply by preparing a placebo identical in appearance to the active agent. However, one study in which the identical appearance of drug and placebo was achieved, but blinding was not, is instructive to review here:

Example. In the early 1970s, healthy adults were enrolled in an experimental study in which they were asked to take either vitamin C (3 g/day) or a lactose placebo for 9 months, during which time the incidence of colds was monitored (Karlowski et al., 1975). Because during the follow-up period some subjects indicated that they were biting into and tasting the preparation that they had been given, the investigators asked all subjects at the conclusion of the study to guess the group to which they had been assigned. Of the 102 who attempted a guess, 79 were correct (77%). The following table summarizes the incidence of colds in persons assigned to each of the two treatment groups, as well as in the subgroup of subjects who guessed incorrectly:

Treatment guessed	Treatment received	No. of subjects	No. with ≥2 colds
Vitamin C	Placebo	11	2 (18%)
—	Vitamin C	101	36 (36%)
Placebo	Vitamin C	12	8 (67%)
—	Placebo	89	42 (47%)

In the group assigned to receive placebo, there was an overall excess (47% vs. 36%) in the percentage of subjects with two or more colds. However, a larger difference was associated with a subject's believing he or she was assigned to a particular group: 36% of subjects assigned to receive vitamin C had two or more colds, twice the incidence in persons who, though they actually were taking placebo, thought they were taking vitamin C. A similar difference was found for persons receiving the vitamin but believing it was a placebo—their incidence was higher than persons receiving placebo (67% vs. 47%). Since a subject's suspicion of the group to which he or she had been assigned so strongly influenced the results, and since a subject's suspicion was much more often right than wrong, the validity of the vitamin C–placebo comparison was seriously compromised.

ASSIGNMENT OF SUBJECTS TO TREATMENT GROUPS

How Should the Assignment Be Made?

Any method of patient assignment is acceptable if it guarantees that chance alone dictates the assignment of a particular patient to a particular treatment group. Thus, the more rigid is the process (e.g., the use of a table of random numbers), the better. The provider of care, having made the decision to ask the patient to participate in the study, should have no role in the assignment process. It is necessary to safeguard against letting the provider's judgment as to which patient needs or does not need the therapy under study influence the treatment assignment. Thus, schemes that call simply for alternate assignment of patients to different groups have the potential for bias, at least if it can happen that more than one patient is to be assigned to the groups at the same time.

When Should the Random Assignment Take Place?

In most experimental trials, subjects are assigned to the treatment groups only after they have been informed of the nature of the study and of the therapies they may be offered. For example, in the trial designed to evaluate the efficacy of coronary artery bypass surgery (Principal Investigators of CASS and Associates, 1981), patients who were deemed eligible for surgery, but not those in whom surgery was deemed essential, were asked to allow themselves to be assigned at random to receive the surgery or the medical therapy. The study included only those patients who agreed to submit to the luck of the draw. See Figure 4-1 for a schematic representation of this approach.

There are some circumstances, however, in which it might be advisable to make the random assignment prior to requesting participation ("prerandomization").

1. The investigator and/or clinical collaborators may be uncomfortable with the idea of presenting the possibility of a choice of therapy to a patient. In the case of a life-threatening illness, for example, cancer, perhaps the investigator is concerned that patients not assigned to the newest, most radical measures may withdraw from the trial, even after consent has been given, in order to actively seek these treatments. In such a circumstance, the investigator can randomly assign patients to

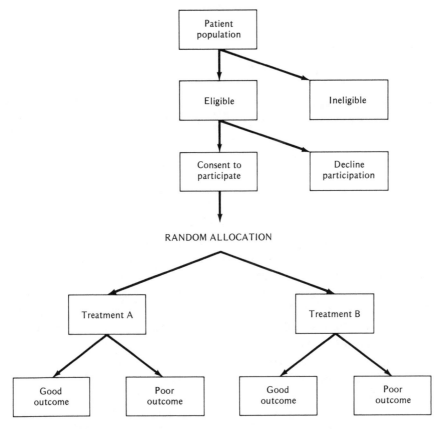

Figure 4-1. Schematic representation of a trial using random allocation of patients to treatment groups.

alternative therapies and either (a) seek consent to participate in the study from all patients, whether they have been assigned the standard or the new therapy (Ellenberg, 1984) or (b) seek consent only from patients assigned the new therapy (Zelen, 1979).

2. Sometimes the efficacy of an intervention is to be studied within a large, defined group of individuals (e.g., members of a prepaid health care plan) who have not actively sought care from the investigative team. This situation might arise in an evaluation of vaccine efficacy in healthy individuals or of a screening technique for cancer. In such situations, it could prove logistically difficult and unnecessarily costly to contact and explain the study to all persons, rather than to just the fraction to whom the intervention measure will be offered.

In order for prerandomization to succeed in evaluating efficacy, a high proportion of subjects to whom the treatment is offered will have to accept it. This is because patients who refuse the treatment must, for analytic purposes, be retained in the same group as those who comply. Therefore, a low level of compliance will obscure any true treatment-related benefit.

In the "conventional" type of experimental study (i.e., agreement to participate prior to randomization), it may be desirable to postpone randomization of a patient until his or her compliance can be evaluated (assuming noncompliance is a possibility, e.g., in a drug or life-style intervention study). The measurement of compliance can take many forms (pill counts, biochemical tests, etc.), but the goal is the same, that is, to eliminate before the start of the study patients who have a high likelihood of not adhering to the regimen offered and who are likely to be a source of misclassification within the study. With this in mind, the study of the value of lowering blood pressure conducted within the Veterans Administration (Veterans Administration Cooperative Study Group on Antihypertensive Agents, 1967) administered to all eligible hypertensive subjects a placebo tablet that contained 5 mg of riboflavin for 2 to 4 months. Because the urine of persons who take riboflavin is fluorescent yellow under ultraviolet light, the investigators had an objective measure of compliance available only to them. Only those subjects whose compliance achieved a designated level—a bare majority of the potential subjects—were enrolled in that randomized trial of antihypertensive agents.

Under What Circumstances Can a Subject Serve as His or Her Own Control?

There are many conditions that affect more than one part of the body, and for some of these conditions it is possible to administer therapy locally that has no effect on untreated lesions elsewhere. In such a situation, it is appropriate to design a study so that one or more lesions are randomly selected for treatment, with others serving as control sites. Such a design has been used to evaluate measures intended to control diabetic retinopathy (Diabetic Retinopathy Study Research Group, 1981) and a number of dermatologic lesions (Gilchrest et al., 1979).

Studies of the efficacy of therapies intended to reduce the frequency or severity of chronic, recurrent problems, such as seizures, arthritic pain, or menopausal hot flashes, can be more precise in a statistical sense if the subject can serve as his or her own control. By evaluating the same subject at different times, in the presence and the absence of the therapy under study, the variability among subjects in the frequency or severity of the problem will not blur true differences in efficacy. This can be achieved experimentally in a "crossover" design, in which the study subjects are divided into two groups and dealt with as shown in Figure 4-2.

At the end of the study, the primary comparison is between, for each subject, the frequency and/or severity of the condition at time-points 1 and 3 (Hills and Armitage, 1979). Events occurring during the period between time-points 1 and 2, the length of which is determined largely by the amount of time needed for the effects of the measures initially administered to dissipate, are not included in the analysis. (Crossover studies are not appropriate for evaluating the efficacy of therapeutic measures whose effects following discontinuation do not dissipate relatively quickly, that is, within several days.)

In crossover studies it is important to include both sequences, therapy–control and control–therapy, for the effect of the therapy can be confounded by the sequence in which it is given (Louis et al., 1984). An example of what could happen if only one sequence is

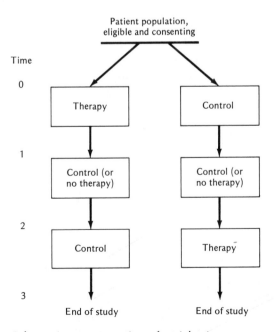

Figure 4-2. Schematic representation of a trial using a crossover design.

used can be seen in a crossover study of estrogen versus placebo for the relief of symptoms associated with the menopause (Coope et al., 1975). Women entering the study averaged 50 to 60 episodes of hot flashes per week. In the group assigned to receive placebo first, the rate fell to 20 per week after 3 months, and fell further, to less than five per week, at the end of a subsequent 3-month period on estrogen therapy. So, in women who started with placebo and crossed over to estrogens, there was evidence of efficacy of estrogen use, although not of an overly great magnitude relative to the "efficacy" of a placebo. It was in the group of women assigned to the other sequence—estrogen first, placebo second—that a large difference occurred. After 3 months on estrogens the frequency of hot flashes fell to less than five per week, but the switch to placebo resulted in a return to the original 50 to 60 per week. While the reasons for the difference in measured efficacy between the two sequences are not well understood, the fact that such a difference can occur reinforces the idea that both possible sequences in a crossover study must be examined.

ASSESSMENT OF ENDPOINTS IN STUDY SUBJECTS

It goes without saying that the vigor with which members of the treatment groups are followed must be equivalent, so that the detection of any study endpoints that do occur is comparable among groups. There should be standard criteria by which the endpoints can be assessed, preferably stipulated at the start of the trial. And, if possible, the person (or persons) who applies the criteria to a particular case should be ignorant of the treatment group to which that case has been assigned.

COMPARISON OF THE TREATMENT GROUPS FOR THE OCCURRENCE OF ENDPOINTS

Which Endpoints to Count

In planning most experimental studies, the choice of endpoint is clear. A study of an analgesic would measure the patient's perception of pain, a study of an antibiotic would measure the disappearance of infection and its clinical manifestations. However, some therapies have such a high potential for serious adverse effects that a broad range of endpoints must be considered. In an experimental study of the efficacy of transplantation in prolonging life, it would not make sense to look at mortality rates in transplanted and non-transplanted patients only for the cause of death at which the therapy was directed (e.g., renal failure, leukemia). Rather, it would be necessary to count causes of death that are related to rejection of the transplant as well. In practice, one probably would tabulate all causes of death combined.

In studies with mortality as an endpoint, a problem arises when the cause of death against which the therapy is directed does not constitute an overwhelming majority of the total deaths, and yet there is no good information available a priori as to which other causes might be affected. The problem exists because neither of the possible comparisons that can be made, rate of therapy-directed causes or rate of all causes, is wholly satisfactory. With the latter comparison, by incorporating many extraneous endpoints, one runs the risk of diluting a true effect of the therapy and making it harder to identify (Sackett and Gent, 1979). With the former comparison, only an incomplete picture of the therapy's effects may be seen. Proper interpretation of such a study requires that both comparisons be made:

Example. A randomized controlled trial was conducted in which clofibrate or a placebo was given for an average of 5.3 years to hypercholesterolemic men in order to influence the incidence and mortality of arteriosclerotic vascular disease (Committee of Principal Investigators, 1978). The rate of nonfatal myocardial infarction was decreased in the clofibrate-treated men, although the rate of fatal heart attack was similar in the two groups. However, other causes of death were more common in the treated group, particularly deaths from digestive diseases and cancer, so that the overall mortality in clofibrate and placebo groups, respectively, was 2.2 and 1.7 per 1,000 per year.

Some conditions that one is attempting to treat or prevent from occurring have measurable antecedents. For example, following treatment for cancer, a death from that cancer is usually preceded by tumor recurrence or metastasis. Death from ventricular arrhythmia following myocardial infarction is often preceded by nonfatal episodes of ventricular arrhythmia. Since one of the factors limiting the power of an experimental study is the number of endpoints, and since these antecedent conditions often occur more commonly than do the endpoints themselves, the monitoring and analysis of these antecedents should increase the statistical power per subject enrolled.

As an investigator, you would be pleased to accept this increase in power as long as the analysis of the occurrence of such an antecedent condition is giving you, qualitatively, the same "answer" as would a study of a larger number of subjects in which the endpoint itself was measured. You will get the same answer to the extent that the occurrence of the antecedent condition is highly predictive of the endpoint:

> *Example.* De Silva et al. (1981) pooled data from six experimental studies of lidocaine prophylaxis in patients with acute myocardial infarction. The incidence of in-hospital ventricular fibrillation (VF) in the group that received lidocaine (16 of 517) was only about one-half the incidence in the group that did not (29 of 505). Deaths due to VF were too uncommon for a meaningful analysis. Nonetheless, since the occurrence of VF following myocardial infarction is a strong risk factor for cardiac death (Ribner et al., 1979), an interim conclusion as to the efficacy of lidocaine prophylaxis in preventing death from VF seems justified.

The following is an example of an intervention that was successful in modifying a suspected antecedent of an endpoint but that turned out to have no influence on the endpoint itself. It should serve as a caution in interpreting experimental studies that measure a therapy's effect on an antecedent alone.

> *Example.* To determine whether the incidence of hepatitis B infection could be reduced in persons undergoing long-term hemodialysis, a large, randomized controlled trial ($n = 1,311$) of hepatitis B vaccine was initiated (Stevens et al., 1984). Active production of antibody to hepatitis B surface antigen (anti-HBs) occurred in about 50% of the vaccinated group and in only 2% of those given a placebo. Nonetheless, during the 25-month follow-up period the incidence of hepatitis B infection in the two groups was nearly identical. The authors concluded that "although anti-HBs is traditionally used as an index of immunity to [hepatitis B] infections, it may not be the crucial protective factor. . . . The vaccine we used may have failed to induce such protective responses in immuno-compromised patients, resulting in our inability to demonstrate its efficacy, even when there appeared to be an appropriate anti-HBs response."

Control of the Potentially Distorting Influence of Other Variables

The University Group Diabetes Project (UGDP) was an experimental trial of the ability of hypoglycemic agents to reduce the occurrence of complications of diabetes. One group of patients was assigned, at random, to receive the drug tolbutamide. These patients happened to differ from those who received no active agent in several respects (e.g., age) so that, apart from any influence of the drug, the tolbutamide therapy group would have been expected to have a somewhat higher rate of complications (Committee for the Assessment of Biometric Aspects of Controlled Trials of Hypoglycemic Agents, 1975).

This sort of imbalance can occur even in an experimental study. It is important to remember that, with respect to other relevant characteristics, randomization merely assures that *on the average* there will be equality of the groups being compared. In any one trial, between-group differences in characteristics related to the study outcome can and do occur (e.g., in the UGDP study), although rarely are they of any great magnitude.

Two strategies are commonly used to prevent the true measure of efficacy of a therapy from being distorted (confounded) in this way:

1. It is possible to form subgroups ("blocks") of subjects who are homogeneous for the presence or level of risk factors for the study outcome, and then to allocate a fixed proportion of the subjects within each block to each of the various treatments. For example, in the study of coronary artery bypass surgery (Principal Investigators of CASS and Associates, 1981) patients were put into groups based on their symptoms, ventricular function, number of diseased vessels, and the institution in which the treatment was being administered. Within each group, equal numbers were assigned to receive medical therapy and surgery, the order of the assignment being selected at random by the study's statisticians.

This procedure guarantees that treatment groups will be comparable with respect to the factor(s) that define the subgroups. The drawback of the strategy is the added complexity at the time of assignment to the treatment groups, and so it is usually reserved for only those characteristics that are expected to have a strong bearing on the study outcome.

2. When the study has been concluded, the treatment groups can be compared for all characteristics believed to have an influence on the outcome. For those characteristics that differ among the groups, it will be possible to control analytically for their interfering effect, either through adjustment (see Appendix) or through other statistical means. In the UGDP study, for example, the difference in mortality from cardiovascular disease between subjects assigned to receive tolbutamide and those assigned receive placebo, an excess of 13.2 per 1,000 per year in the tolbutamide treatment group, was due in part to the higher mean age of the tolbutamide-treated

group. The difference fell to 12.4 per 1,000 per year once the age distributions of the two groups were "forced" to be the same by an adjustment procedure.

Handling Those Subjects Who Were Assigned to One Mode of Therapy But Who Did Not Receive It

Studies vary regarding the frequency with which their subjects, once randomized, fail to receive fully the treatment to which they have been assigned. It is the rare study in which the original assignments are adhered to perfectly. The reason for a change in therapy may be physician-initiated: Perhaps the condition of a patient assigned to the medical arm of a study of coronary artery surgery worsens and the physician feels that surgery is necessary. Or, perhaps a patient develops an adverse reaction to a study drug and the physician must discontinue it. Alternatively, failure to adhere to the prescribed regimen can be due simply to patient noncompliance.

In theory, when analyzing the results of an experimental study there are two possible ways of dealing with patients who did not receive or complete the intended course of therapy: (a) keep them in the groups to which they were originally assigned, thus retaining the experimental nature of the design, and accept the resulting misclassification of patients in terms of treatment actually received; and (b) allow them to "transfer" to the therapy they actually received (or to withdraw from the study altogether), losing the experimental nature of the design but reducing the amount of misclassification that would occur in option (a).

In practice, the first approach (keeping the originally assigned groups) is the one to rely on. Categorizing patients on the basis of therapy received allows for the possibility of "selection" bias to appear, that is, are there characteristics of persons who did not receive or complete the originally assigned therapy that also are correlated with the outcome being measured? Based on what we know about the reasons for changes in therapy following randomization, and on the characteristics and outcomes of patients who do change therapies, a considerable amount of selection bias would be expected to result in most studies. For instance, there are therapies that, if effective, are expected to produce demonstrable improvement in the patient's status before the full course of therapy is finished. It would be expected that patients who do not complete the full course will be disproportionately numerous in the group assigned to the therapy that is truly less effective. In such situations, the elimination of patients with an incomplete course of therapy from the analysis will diminish the measured efficacy of the superior therapy.

Even when the outcome does not influence compliance in such a direct way, the failure to maintain originally assigned groups can lead to a biased result. An instructive example comes from an experimental study in which, in an effort to reduce cardiac mortality, the drug clofibrate (which lowers the concentration of serum cholesterol) or a placebo was prescribed to patients who had sustained a myocardial infarction (Coronary Drug Project Research Group, 1980). During the 5-year period of the study, adherence to the prescribed regimen was monitored in both treatment and placebo groups. The cumulative mortality was found not to differ between the clofibrate and placebo treatment groups. However, no matter which regimen had been prescribed, those who adhered to it (80% or more of the time) experienced a mortality of about 15%, whereas the mortality in persons who were less compliant was about 27%. If, in the analysis, the investigators had placed the noncompliant clofibrate patients into the placebo group, they would have found a spurious benefit associated with use of the drug.

Statistical Analysis of Experimental Studies

The topic of statistical anaysis lies outside the scope of this book. An excellent introduction to the subject, one that emphasizes practical aspects and provides examples, can be found in an article by Peto et al. (1977).

LIMITATIONS OF EXPERIMENTAL STUDIES OF THERAPEUTIC EFFICACY

Randomized controlled trials generally are not cheap to conduct. A considerable expenditure of resources is required to assemble a group of subjects and to monitor them over time. There are also substantial administrative costs associated with the multiinstitutional collaboration that is often required. Since the magnitude of the cost is in part related to the number of subjects studied, there are usually financial restrictions on the size of most experimental studies.

Of course, the smaller the number of subjects, the smaller will be the power of the trial to reliably determine the difference between treatment groups (see Appendix). The following illustrates the ambiguities in interpretation that can arise when a seemingly large study is not quite large enough:

Example. During the mid- to late 1970s, a collaborative investigative group wished to determine whether patients with cutaneous melanoma would benefit from chemotherapy, immunotherapy, or both, after resection of tumor (Veronesi et al., 1982). They randomly assigned 761 patients at high risk of tumor recurrence, based on depth of skin invasion or the presence of regional node involvement, to one of four treatment groups: (1) surgery alone; (2) surgery followed by intravenous dacarbazine administration; (3) surgery followed by immunotherapy with bacille Calmette-Guérin (BCG) vaccine; and (4) surgery followed by both dacarbazine and BCG administration. The survival at 3 years among members of each group was as follows:

Treatment group	3-year survival	Difference from surgery alone
Surgery alone	41.6%	—
Surgery + dacarbazine	46.5%	4.9%
Surgery + BCG	48.7%	7.1%
Surgery + dacarbazine + BCG	50.0%	8.4%

The difference in survival between the group that received surgery alone and each of the others was quite compatible with there being no true difference, that is, each of the three p values was large. The authors concluded that "an advantage of adjuvant treatment was not demonstrated. Either a difference did not exist, or it was of limited clinical importance."

So, what are you, as a physician, to do for the patient whose melanoma and positive regional lymph nodes have recently been resected? A difference in 3-year survival of 5 to 8% may be "of limited clinical importance" relative to the initial hopes of these investigators, but you do not want to deprive *your* patients of an extra chance of survival of that magnitude: For most of them, that extra chance is probably worth the costs and adverse effects of the chemotherapy and/or immunotherapy. And yet, despite the fact that the results are based on the study of 761 patients, a larger number than in most clinical trials, there is a reasonable probability that the improved survival in the groups that received one of the supplementary therapies was simply the result of chance. *Differences in efficacy between treatment regimens that are of clinical importance often cannot be resolved in clinical trials because of the trial's inability to enroll enough patients.*

Figure 4-3 depicts the number of subjects (n) needed in each of

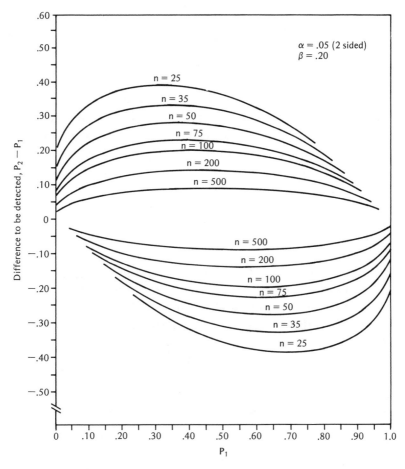

Figure 4-3. Sample sizes required for testing two independent proportions, P_1 and P_2, with 80% probability of obtaining a significant result at the 5% (two-sided) level. n = Number of observations *per group*. (Adapted from P. Feigl: A graphical aid for determining sample size when comparing two independent proportions. Department of Biostatistics, Technical Report No. 6, University of Washington, Seattle, July 1977.)

two groups of equal size to reliably (80% of the time) detect a significant difference among them (at $P = 0.05$). The number is related to (a) the frequency with which the study endpoint occurs in one of the groups (P_1, ranging from 0 to 1.0) and (b) the true difference between the frequency of the study endpoint in the two groups ($P_2 - P_1$, ranging from −0.5 to 0.6). So, for example, if 30% of patients with a given condition show symptomatic improvement after treatment with a placebo, and if in truth 50% treated with drug

A improve ($P_2 - P_1 = 0.50 - 0.30 = 0.20$), then it will require slightly fewer than 200 patients (slightly fewer than 100 per group) to reliably identify this difference. Note that for between-group differences smaller than 0.10, several hundred or more patients per treatment group are needed. The smaller the benefit of the therapy being evaluated, the larger is the study required to determine it.

Because of the limited power of most clinical trials to determine clinically important differences between two therapeutic regimens, it is only under unusual circumstances (e.g., a very large number of subjects relative to that needed to detect the differences expected) that the patient population should be split into three or more groups. There will be strong temptations to form these additional groups. For example, there may be several promising therapies, for example, dacarbazine and BCG for melanoma. Or, there may be some uncertainty as to the proper dose/duration of a single therapy, and it might seem advantageous to try several. Indeed, after a recent clinical trial in which aspirin was found not to lower the risk of recurrence in persons with a previous myocardial infarction (Aspirin Myocardial Infarction Study Research Group, 1980), some evidence has been accumulated to indicate that a beneficial effect might have been present had only a different dose of aspirin been used (Lorenz et al., 1984). Nonetheless, obtaining an adequate number of subjects to provide a valid test of at least one hypothesis should remain the first priority and, as indicated above, that number is often large.

QUESTIONS, CHAPTER 4

4-1. The following is paraphrased from an article published several years ago on the evaluation of the efficacy of a group of drugs:

We do not discuss randomized controlled trials of these drugs because our concern has been to evaluate the effects of the drugs on populations rather than on individuals. Thus, although randomized controlled trials provide unique information on the effects of drugs, they would concern us only if the study groups were representative of defined subgroups of the general population. Such representation is rarely possible in these trials, which generally involve volunteers.

You disagree with the opinion expressed above. Why?

4-2. After obtaining informed consent, 100 patients with cancer X were randomly assigned to one of two therapeutic regimens, surgery or chemotherapy. It turned out that while all 50 patients assigned to chemotherapy received their treatment, 14 of the 50 assigned to receive surgery did not: Five became too ill between the date of randomization and the scheduled date of surgery, and nine had second thoughts and declined to have the operation. However, all of these 14 were offered, and they accepted, chemotherapy. The survival of all patients was monitored for 1 year.

In comparing the relative efficacy of the two therapeutic regimens, which patient groups should be compared? Why?

ANSWERS

4-1. Randomized controlled trials always involve volunteers, so there will always be a need to generalize to a reference population that is not entirely similar to the study population; the former will contain potential nonvolunteers as well. The alternative approaches to evaluating drug efficacy, however—one or other of the nonexperimental designs—have a potentially more important drawback: Patients who receive and do not receive the drug are likely to have inherently different risks of the outcome that the therapy seeks to prevent.

So, in our search for internally valid studies we pay particular attention to the results of experimental studies, and we certainly do not eschew them. The process of generalizing to a reference population may still be tricky, but it cannot even be begun until there is confidence that the comparison among the study subjects themselves has some validity.

4-2. The survival of the 50 patients originally assigned to receive chemotherapy should be compared with that of the 50 patients originally assigned to undergo surgery. If these groups are not preserved in the analysis, and the analysis is based instead on therapy received (or on an analysis that deletes the "crossover" patients altogether), a biased comparison could easily emerge. The patients assigned to undergo surgery but who did not do so may be quite atypical with respect to survival (note that five such patients were too ill). Failure to keep them in the surgery group would probably make surgical therapy appear efficacious in the treatment of cancer X in the absence of any true difference between results for surgical therapy and chemotherapy.

REFERENCES

Aspirin Myocardial Infarction Study Research Group: A randomized controlled trial of aspirin in persons recovered from myocardial infarction. *JAMA* 1980; 243:661–669.

Cobb LA, Thomas GI, Dillard DH, et al.: An evaluation of internal-mammary artery ligation by a double-blind technic. *N Engl J Med* 1959; 260:1115–1118.

Committee for the Assessment of Biometric Aspects of Controlled Trials of Hypoglcemic Agents: *JAMA* 1975; 231:583–608.

Committee of Principal Investigators: A co-operative trial in the primary prevention of ischaemic heart disease using clofibrate. *Br Heart J* 1978; 40:1069–
1118.

Coope J, Thomson JM, Poller L: Effects of "natural estrogen" replacement therapy
on menopausal symptoms and blood clotting. *Br Med J* 1975; 4:139–143.

Coronary Drug Project Research Group: Aspirin in coronary heart disease. *J Chron
Dis* 1976; 29:625–642.

Coronary Drug Project Research Group: Influence of adherence to treatment and
response of cholesterol on mortality in the coronary drug project. *N Engl J
Med* 1980; 303:1038–1041.

Dayton S, Pearce ML, Hashimoto S, et al.: A controlled clinical trial of a diet high
in unsaturated fat in preventing complications of atherosclerosis. *Circulation*
1969; 39–40 (suppl 2):1–63.

DeSilva RA, Hennekens CH, Lown B, et al.: Lignocaine prophylaxis in acute myocardial infarction: An evaluation of randomised trials. *Lancet* 1981; 2:855–
858.

Diabetic Retinopathy Study Research Group: Photocoagulation treatment of pro-
liferative diabetic retinopathy: Clinical appication of diabetic retinopathy
study (DRS) findings. DRS Report Number 8. *Ophthalmology* 1981; 88:583–
600.

Ellenberg SS: Randomization designs in comparative clinical trials. *N Engl J Med*
1984; 310:1404–1408.

Gilchrest BA, Rowe JW, Brown RS, et al.: Ultraviolet phototherapy of uremic pru-
ritus: Long-term results and possible mechanism of action. *Ann Intern Med*
1979; 91:17–21.

Hills M, Armitage P: The two-period cross-over clinical trial. *Br J Clin Pharmacol*
1979; 8:7–20.

Hypertension Detection and Follow-up Program Cooperative Group: Five-year
findings of the Hypertension Detection and Follow-up Program: I. Reduction in mortality of persons with high blood pressure, including mild hypertension. *JAMA* 1979a; 242:2562–2571.

Hypertension Detection and Follow-up Program Cooperative Group. Five-year
findings of the Hypertension Detection and Follow-up Program: II. Mortality by race-sex and age. *JAMA* 1979b; 242:2572–2577.

Javid MJ, Nordby EJ, Ford LT, et al.: Safety and efficacy of chymopapain (Chy-
modiactin) in herniated nucleus pulposus with sciatica: Results of a randomized, double-blind study. *JAMA* 1983; 249:2489–2494.

Karlowski TR, Chalmers TC, Frenkel LD, et al.: Ascorbic acid for the common
cold: A prophylactic and therapeutic trial. *JAMA* 1975; 231:1038–1042.

Lipid Research Clinics Program: The Lipid Research Clinics coronary primary prevention trial results. *JAMA* 1984; 251:351–364.

Lorenz RL, Weber M, Kotzur J, et al.: Improved aortocoronary bypass patency by
low-dose aspirin (100 mg daily): Effects on platelet aggregation and throm-
boxane formation. *Lancet* 1984; 1:1261–1264.

Louis TA, Lavori PW, Bailar JC, et al.: Crossover and self-controlled designs in
clinical research. *N Engl J Med* 1984; 310:24–31.

Mitchell JRA: Blood pressure and mortality in the very old. *Lancet* 1983; 2:1248.

Peto R, Pike MC, Armitage NE, et al.: Design and analysis of randomized clinical trials requiring prolonged observation of each patient: II. Analysis and examples. *Br J Cancer* 1977; 35:1–39.

Principal Investigators of CASS and Associates: The National Heart, Lung, and Blood Institute coronary artery surgery study. *Circulation* 1981; 63(suppl 1):I1–I81.

Ribner HS, Isaacs ES, Frishman WH: Lidocaine prophylaxis against ventricular fibrillation in acute myocardial infarction. *Progr Cardiovasc Dis* 1979; 21:287–313.

Sackett DL, Gent M: Controversy in counting and attributing events in clinical trials *N Engl J Med* 1979; 301:1410–1412.

Shapiro S, Strax P, Venet L: Periodic breast cancer screening in reducing mortality from breast cancer. *JAMA* 1971; 215:1777–1785.

Stevens CE, Alter HJ, Taylor PE, et al.: Hepatitis B vaccine in patients receiving hemodialysis: Immunogenicity and efficacy. *N Engl J Med* 1984; 311:496–500.

Veronesi U, Adamus J, Abuert C, et al.: A randomized trial of adjuvant chemotherapy and immunotherapy in cutaneous melanoma. *N Engl J Med* 1982; 307:913–916.

Veterans Administration Cooperative Study Group on Antihypertensive Agents: Effects of treatment on morbidity in hypertension: Results in patients with diastolic blood pressures averaging 115 through 129 mm Hg. *JAMA* 1967; 202:116–122.

Zelen M: A new design for randomized clinical trials. *N Engl J Med* 1979; 300:1242–1245.

5 Therapeutic Efficacy: Nonexperimental Studies

Experimental studies are the best method we have of evaluating the efficacy of therapy. Nonetheless, therapeutic decisions often have to be made in the absence of data obtained in this way. Perhaps a therapeutic measure was introduced into the practices of some health care providers at a time when randomized controlled trials were the exception rather than the rule. Perhaps it was a therapeutic measure of a sort that even today often does not undergo evaluation in a randomized trial prior to being widely adopted, for instance, a dietary or environmental manipulation. Or, perhaps a treatment has been tested and found to be modestly effective in a randomized controlled trial but, because of the size of the trial, this result could have arisen simply by chance (see Chapter 4).

CRITERIA FOR THE VALIDITY OF NONEXPERIMENTAL STUDIES

In the absence of decisive experimental data, where can we turn for evidence that will make our therapeutic decision a more rational one? We must make an attempt to exploit the fact that, among patients with the same illness, it is often possible to find groups that happen to be treated in different ways. To evaluate the efficacies of the treatments relative to one another, the experiences of these patient groups following treatment are compared.

Unfortunately, simple comparisons of this sort may be misleading, for the distribution of illness severity may be very different among the groups. Persons with a mild form of an illness often receive different types of treatment than persons with a more severe form. Thus, the measured differences between the experiences of patient groups receiving alternative therapies may have as much or more to do with differences in characteristics of the patients themselves as with differences in the effectiveness of the therapies. For example, a comparison of the survival experience of persons with lung cancer who received (a) surgery followed by radiation therapy or (b) surgery alone would probably be biased in favor of the latter group, since supplemental radiation therapy might be prescribed only for patients with demonstrable metastases, patients with a particularly poor prognosis. Similarly, several series of patients with cirrhosis of the liver and esophageal varices who underwent shunt surgery had a better survival experience than did other cirrhotic patients with demonstrable varices, but this now seems to have been due almost entirely to the poorer condition of the members of the latter group (Sacks et al., 1982).

Furthermore, among patients with a given illness there may be some who have other health problems that proscribe the use of one of several available therapies. For example, the level of comorbidity in patients with end-stage renal disease who receive dialysis therapy is substantially higher than in those who receive cadaveric transplantation (Vollmer et al., 1983). Thus, a comparison of survival in persons receiving these two modes of therapy would spuriously favor the transplant group.

Under what circumstances can data gathered outside randomized controlled trials be used to draw valid inferences concerning the efficacy of therapy? Not everyone offers the same answer to this question! Some say that results from studies in which randomization has not taken place can almost never be trusted, that the factors influencing the selection of certain patients for certain therapies are too strong to be overcome (Sacks et al., 1982). At the other extreme are those who believe that randomized controlled trials are impractical, unnecessary, and often unethical, and who would allow most therapeutic decisions to be based on results obtained in nonexperimental studies (Gehan and Freirich, 1979; Van der Linden, 1980).

The view espoused here is an intermediate one. On the one hand, since we commonly employ the findings of nonexperimental studies in judging what might be done to prevent disease, or to prevent adverse effects of therapy, it seems reasonable that these findings could play at least some role in judging the benefits of therapy.[1] On the other hand, the possibility for bias in using nonexperimental data to judge therapeutic efficacy is great (see above), so it is particularly important to specify the conditions that must prevail in these studies so that the inferences drawn regarding efficacy can be valid.

It goes without saying that, at minimum, a valid comparison between two or more treatment groups requires monitoring the course of the illness under treatment similarly among the groups. Whether the tools for monitoring are questionnaires, laboratory values, or death records, the same tools must be applied in the same way for all subjects in order for the study's findings to be credible.

A second criterion for validity, typically much more difficult to achieve than the one just mentioned, requires that at least one of two conditions must hold: (a) The size of the observed difference in outcome among the treatment groups substantially exceeds that which could be expected on the basis of inherent differences among the groups with respect to other characteristics that influence the outcome of illness (e.g., illness severity), and (b) The differences among the various treatment groups, with respect to other factors that influence the outcome of illness, can be made sufficiently small (by means of appropriately matching subjects in the groups and/or making adjustments in the analysis) so as not to interfere with the evaluation of the influence of treatment per se.

Here are two examples in which the first condition appears to have been met.

Example. A group of physicians performed bone marrow transplantation in 24 children who had relapsed after an initial course of chemotherapy for acute lymphoblastic leukemia (Johnson et al., 1981). At the end of a mean follow-up period of about 2 years, 11 children were alive (9 in remission), in contrast to only 2 of 21 (1 in remission) children who had relapsed but received only chemotherapy additionally. The children had not been randomly assigned to the two treatment groups; rather, those who had an HLA-identical donor available were offered marrow transplantation; the others were not. There is no reason to believe that the availability of an HLA-identical donor correlates much, if at all, with survival in this disease. Thus, it is very likely that the difference in survival is almost entirely the result of a difference in the efficacy of the two therapeutic approaches.

---

[1]For Example, there are virtually no data from randomized controlled trials that have contributed to our conclusions that lung cancer could be prevented by not smoking cigarettes, or that vaginal adenocarcinoma could be prevented by avoiding prenatal exposure to diethylstilbestrol (DES).

Example. Monson et al. (1973) followed 353 women treated for Stage I endo-metrial cancer at a single Boston hospital. Those who received radiation therapy after hysterectomy had a significantly greater 5-year survival than did those who had hysterectomy only. The face that his difference occurred despite an initially poorer life expectancy (on the basis of tumor grade) in the irradiated group argues strongly for the efficacy of post-hysterectomy irradiation in this condition.

Other investigators have started with treatment groups of inher-ently different prognoses but, by identifying important prognostic characteristics and by matching or adjusting for them, they were able to achieve a fair degree of between-group comparability (i.e., their studies met the second condition for validity).

Example. To evaluate the efficacy of lidocaine prophylaxis in preventing death following acute myocardial infarction, the outcome of patients hospitalized with a myocardial infarction was monitored (Horwitz and Feinstein, 1981). In com-paring the survival of patients who did and did not receive lidocaine prophy-laxis, the investigators noted that some patients had ventricular tachycardia or other ventricular ectopic activity, conditions that mandated the use of lidocaine. Because these abnormalities are strongly predictive of mortality, inclusion of these patients in the analysis would bias the study toward finding a deleterious effect of lidocaine. Accordingly, the investigators chose to "match" on the absence of the above characteristics by eliminating all such patients from the study. (They also matched the groups being compared on other factors less strongly related with risk of mortality—age, sex, race, and date of hospitalization.)

Example. A regional center for the treatment of end-stage renal disease evalu-ated the mortality experience of its patients (Vollmer et al., 1983). The initial comparison showed that patients who had received a cadaveric transplant had 58% of the mortality of those who had received dialysis. However, the investi-gators at the center observed that several characteristics associated with high mortality (e.g., hypertension or diabetes as the cause of the renal failure, and the presence of concurrent illness) were present to a greater extent in patients in the dialysis group. When the confounding influence of these variables was controlled (see Chapter 8), the difference in mortality between transplant and dialysis groups was eliminated.

Example. In designing a study to evaluate the efficacy of a vaccine against pneu-mococcal pneumonia, investigators at the Centers for Disease Control were con-fronted with the problem that persons to whom the vaccine was being given— the elderly, persons with an immune disorder, and so on—were at far higher risk of contracting the disease than were other persons. Thus, a simple compar-ison of disease rates in vaccinated and unvaccinated persons would be likely to seriously underestimate the efficacy of the vaccine. (A randomized controlled trial to evaluate this issue could be logistically difficult and extremely expensive to conduct. The recruitment of potential subjects, their follow-up for the occur-rence of pneumonia, and the low rate of the disease are obstacles that have prevented such a study from being undertaken in the United States).To deal with this problem, the investigators (Broome et al., 1981) took advantage of the fact that there are a number of types of *P. pneumoniae* and that the vaccine is directed at only a minority of them. So, among persons with pneumococcal pneumonia they identified some in whom vaccine-type organisms were cultured and others in whom nonvaccine-type organisms were cultured. Since there was no reason to believe that the two groups were different in their underlying risk of contracting penumococcal pneumonia, a comparison of vaccination histories between the two could be expected to provide a valid estimate of efficacy.

Comparisons of Concurrent and Nonconcurrent Patient Groups

As a means of increasing between-group comparability, it is tempting to compare the outcomes of patients treated in one way during a recent time period with those of patients treated in another way in the past. On the surface, an evaluation of this sort would appear to have much to recommend it: In many situations, a greater degree of similarity (in terms of prognostic factors) should be present between two groups of patients being treated at different times than between two groups seen at the same time but who receive different therapies. However, unless the difference in outcome between the groups is substantial, the results of such evaluations are difficult to interpret, for characteristics relevant to the study outcome may differ in recent and not-so-recent patients. For example, in a 7-year, randomized clinical trial of treatment for cancer of the prostate gland, it was noted that the annual mortality among patients enrolled in the placebo treatment group in the last several years of the trial was lower than that of patients enrolled in that group in the first several years (Veterans Administration Cooperative Urological Research Group, 1967). Thus, had this not been an experimental study, and had placebo been replaced by an active therapy in the later time period, an apparent benefit associated with that therapy would have been seen, in the absence of any true effect on survival.

Even if an attempt is made to measure and adjust for these patient characteristics (see Question 5-2), it may not be possible to measure comparably some important ones (e.g., disease severity) in the various time periods, either because of changes in the nature of patient records or because the methods of evaluating patients have changed over time.

Finally, problems in interpretation can be introduced by the fact that ways of caring for patients with a given condition often consist of more than a single measure, and that these other ways ("supportive care") may change over time as well. So, even if it is felt that there has been a true change in the prognosis of patients with a particular disorder, it may be difficult to ascribe that change to a specific therapeutic agent.

Nonetheless, a big difference in outcome between groups treated in different ways in not widely spaced periods of time should not be ignored. For example, of 325 Rh(D)-negative women who received two 100-μg doses of anti-D immunoglobulin in the third trimester of their first pregnancy and another dose at delivery if their infant was Rh(D)-positive, only 2 developed anti-D antibodies in a subsequent Rh(D)-positive pregnancy (Tovey et al., 1983). In contrast, based on the experience of Rh(D)-negative women from the same region, pregnant in the 2 preceding years and who were treated only at delivery, 17.9 women in the more recent group would have been expected to develop antibodies. Since little else of consequence had changed with regard to the management of these women, it seems hard to dispute the efficacy of the antenatal prophylaxis.

Obtaining Comparable Numerators and Denominators Between Treatment Groups

Whether the comparison group of patients is concurrent or historical, a strategy to aid in choosing comparable treatment groups is to identify, if possible, a point in the disease process at which the decision to use the treatment would generally be made. The groups would be defined on the basis of treatment initiated at that time (and could include a group that received no treatment if present). The various groups would be compared from that time forward for the development of disease progression/complications, and retained in those groups even if the therapy were altered subsequently.

For example, in a nonexperimental study attempting to evaluate the efficacy of coronary artery bypass surgery, one might identify patients who had undergone their first coronary angiography, some of whom subsequently received surgery (within a predefined time following angiography) and the rest not. The two groups would be compared for, say, mortality from heart disease starting at the time the decision was made to perform surgery and at the equivalent time after angiography for nonsurgical cases. Bypass surgery in the latter group at a later time would be disregarded (the patients would remain in the nonsurgical group), for their "transfer" to the group that initially received surgery could introduce an important source of bias (see p. 64).

> *Example.* In comparing the case-fatality between patients who were and were not administered lidocaine, investigators (Horwitz and Feinstein, 1981) were concered that some patients died so soon after entry to the hospital that lidocaine could not have been ordered, even had a physician wanted to so so. To include these patients in the analysis would be to severely bias the results toward finding a beneficial effect associated with lidocaine. Thus, patients who died prior to admission to the hospital's coronary care unit were excluded from the study.

Reminder: Nonexperimental Studies of Efficacy Must Be Interpreted with Caution!

It is easier to stipulate the conditions needed for a nonexperimental study of therapeutic efficacy to provide a valid result—that is, small between-group differences in factors predictive of outcome (confounding factors) either inherently or after manipulation in the study design and/or analysis—than to determine unequivocally if they are present in a given instance. The only times one can be really "sure" that the between-group differences in confounding factors are small are when the results of experimental studies have corroborated those of the nonexperimental studies, and these are just the times that the nonexperimental studies are the least needed.

Let's consider two examples, both of which are intended to keep us from becoming overconfident in our ability to derive valid comparisons from nonexperimental studies, no matter how hard we strive to achieve comparability of treatment groups:

> *Example.* The results of six nonexperimental studies that evaluated the efficacy of anticoagulant drugs in reducing early mortality from acute myocardial infarction were summarized by Sacks et al. (1982). A 17.1% difference in mortality was found (mortality in patients given anticoagulants was 18.0% vs. 35.1% in controls). In four of the studies, data were available on some or all of the following prognostic factors: age, sex, location and severity of infarction, history of previous infarction and other diseases. After adjustment for them, the overall mortality difference favoring the anticoagulant-treated group was reduced to 11.0%. Nonetheless, the pooling of data from 10 randomized controlled trials of anticoagulants in acute myocardial infarction revealed a difference of only 3.9% (still favoring the anticoagulant-treated group). Thus, the adjustment for prognostic factors that were measured in the nonexperimental studies could in part, but not fully, eliminate the confounding due to underlying differences between patients in the anticoagulant-treated and control groups.

Example. In an effort to reduce mortality from lung cancer among men who smoke heavily (one or more packs of cigarettes per day), investigators in Maryland initiated an early detection program (Levin et al. 1982). Subjects (*n* = 10,387) were assigned to one of two intervention groups over a 5-year period: chest x-ray film annually or annual x-ray film accompanied by cytological examination of aerosol-induced sputum (annually) and of spontaneously produced sputum (three times each year). At the study's inception, none of the men were under treatment for lung cancer or suspected lung cancer.

While the primary comparison was between the lung cancer mortality rates in these two groups, it was conceivable that the two interventions were similarly efficacious relative to no screening at all. Thus, the investigators also compared the rates in their subjects with those of male cigarette smokers in whom no systematic screening was done during a prior study of male veterans. The results were as follows:

Group	Annual lung cancer mortality (per 1,000)
x-ray film only	2.8
x-ray film + cytology	2.3
Veterans	1.7*

(*Adjusted to the distribution of age and daily cigarette consumption of the screened subjects.)

Compared with the group offered only the annual x-ray film, the group offered the x-ray film and cytology had a modest reduction in lung cancer mortality, but this could easily have been the result of chance ($P = 0.37$). On the other hand, the "unscreened" male veterans had the lowest rate of all, significantly ($P = 0.05$) different from the rate of either of the screened groups, even after adjustment for a key prognostic variable, the number of cigarettes smoked.

We suspect that the screening programs did not truly produce an increased mortality from lung cancer and, while it is possible that this paradoxical result could have come about from lung cancer deaths in the screened group being more accurately identified and labelled as such on death certificates, it is likely that the incidence of lung cancer in the men who volunteered to be screened was anomalously high. Although men with existing or medically suspected cancers were excluded, it appears that men with symptoms of early cancer or symptoms correlated with development of cancer preferentially enrolled in the screening program.

The notion raised in the preceding examples, that, even after controlling for all measurable, relevant characteristics there could be some hard-to-define characteristic that may vary considerably between the treatment groups—and as a result distort the true difference in the measured efficacy of the therapeutic alternatives—

has at times received explicit consideration. Mossey and Shapiro (1982) classified a random sample of elderly persons with respect to an index of "objective" health status, the index being based on the presence of certain medical conditions (weighted for severity) and on the degree to which the conditions caused the persons to obtain health care services in the prior year. In addition, the subjects were asked the following question: "For your age would you say, in general, your health is excellent, good, fair, poor?" Mortality rates were monitored in this group ($n = 3,128$) for the next 7 years. Persons who reported their health as "poor" had a mortality rate nearly three times that of persons who reported their health as excellent, even after the influence of "objective" health status had been controlled. The message: While these investigators achieved some success, much of the time we are simply not able to measure (and thus not able to control for) some important factors that bear on the outcome of the condition for which we are evaluating the therapeutic choices. As a consequence, without our knowing it, the treatment groups that are formed in the absence of randomization may be at quite different risks of the outcome under study.

INTEGRATING RESULTS FROM NONEXPERIMENTAL STUDIES WITH EXTERNAL DATA

There are relatively few experimental studies in humans to help evaluate whether a suspected factor plays an etiologic role in disease occurrence. It is usually far more feasible to conduct a randomized trial of a potentially therapeutic agent than one of a potentially etiologic agent. Thus, the question of the adequcy of evidence from nonexperimental studies for inferring cause and effect is addressed often by epidemiologists dealing with the causes of disease. What criteria do they use that are relevant to judging, from data gathered in nonexperimental studies, whether (and to what extent) an agent is effective in treating disease? Apart from the two criteria that have been stressed already—the presence of a large difference in outcome between the treatment groups and a small difference in confounding factors—the epidemiologist looks to the plausibility of the cause-and-effect relationship, that is, does it make sense on the basis of other knowledge? Needless to say, the use of this criterion introduces a great deal of subjectivity into the matter, and it is responsible for many disagreements concerning disease etiology, for example air pollution and lung disease, diet and cancer. Still, as hard as it is to apply at times, this criterion cannot be ignored.

Since there is almost always a good reason (pharmacologic, mechanical, nutritional, etc.) for the introduction of most therapeutic measures, the issue of a priori expectation tends to be less useful when applied to therapeutic questions than to etiologic ones. However, not all therapies have uniform effects over time and/or among individuals. The more the pattern of differences in the outcomes associated with alternative therapies corresponds to a priori expectation, the stronger is the case that can be made for true efficacy (Weiss, 1981).

Example. In case-control studies of postmenopausal women with hip and forearm fractures, the prior use of noncontraceptive estrogens was associated with a decrease in risk, but only if the hormones had been taken for 6 or more years and not discontinued prior to the time of the study (Weiss et al., 1980; Paganini-Hill et al., 1981). Earlier studies of bone density had shown a steadily increasing difference between estrogen-treated and control women over a period of several years (Lindsay et al., 1976), but this difference was no longer apparent within a year or two after women had stopped taking the drug (Lindsay et al., 1978). Since the results of the case-control studies "fit" the expectation based on other data, not only as to the overall direction of the effect but to the particulars of duration and recency of use, a strong argument could be made for the efficacy of noncontraceptive estrogens in reducing the incidence of fractures.

Example. Of 11 patients with "intractable" rheumatoid arthritis treated with total lymphoid radiation (2,000 rad), 9 showed improvement in signs and symptoms at the end of a 5- to 18-month period of observation (Kotzin et al., 1981). Although there was no formal comparison group, the credibility of a beneficial effect of this form of therapy is supported by the following: (a) The magnitude of the improvement in symptoms and signs was greater than would have been expected on the basis of observations on "similar" untreated patients. (b) The radiation produced immunosuppression in these patients. Immunosuppression is associated with remission in experimental autoimmune disease. (c) The timing of the symptomatic improvement—no improvement until at least 1 month after irradiation and a maximal response at approximately 6 months—was roughly that to be expected on the basis of an immunosuppressive effect.

While the degree of improvement (and adverse effects) relative to that which would occur following alternative therapeutic measures can hardly be evaluated in a "design" such as this (indeed, the same investigators then initiated a randomized controlled trial comparing total lymphoid irradiation and cytotoxic drugs) the nature of the findings in these 11 patients is sufficiently strong to warrent further evaluation of the therapeutic role of total lymphoid irradiation.

Example. In the study mentioned earlier that sought to measure the effect of prophylactic lidocaine on mortality following myocardial infarction (Horwitz and Feinstein, 1981), the investigators categorized each death as being attributable to an arrhythmia or to other causes. The categorization was done without knowledge of whether lidocaine had been administered to the patient. There was about a three fold reduction in mortality from ventricular arrhythmia in the lidocaine-treated group, whereas mortality from other cardiac causes was identical in the two groups. The restriction of the mortality reduction to a particular cause of death, especially one that would have been predicted prior to the study to be sensitive to the effect of this medication, makes it less likely that the results could be explained by the tendency for lidocaine to be used selectively in low-risk patients.

ACTIONS BASED ON RESULTS OBTAINED IN NONEXPERIMENTAL STUDIES

Once one or more nonexperimental studies of the efficacy of a particular therapy have been completed, there are three general courses of action that a health care provider can take with regard to the therapy:

1. The therapy has been demonstrated to have no or very little effect, and there are no apparent biases to have nullified a true benefit. *Action:* The therapy should not be used.
2. The therapy has been demonstrated to have a great deal of efficacy, far beyond what could reasonably be attributed to possible biases, and this outweighs any known adverse effects. *Action:* The therapy can be put into use (or continue to be used). It is no longer ethical to conduct randomized controlled trials to evaluate the efficacy of this therapy.
3. The therapy has been demonstrated to have some efficacy, but not beyond what could reasonably be attributed to possible biases. The efficacy outweighs any known adverse effects. *Action:* The therapy could be put into use (or could continue to be used) on an interim basis until the results of randomized controlled trials or more definitive nonexperimental studies are available.

Sometimes the choice among these courses of action is clear-cut. For instance, based on the results obtained in the nonexperimental studies presented earlier, it would be hard to dispute the efficacy of bone marrow transplantation in treating acute lymphoblastic leukemia or, in Rh(D)-negative women, of prepartum anti-D immunoglobulin in preventing the development of anti-D antibodies. Thus, most of us would be willing to forgo the requirement of a randomized controlled trial and would not deny either of these therapies to patients for whom they are indicated. In contrast, only the most uncritical would accept as definitive the uncontrolled study of lymph node irradiation for rheumatoid arthritis, and there would be wide support for an experimental trial to evaluate this measure.

Often the appropriate course of action is less clear. A therapy can appear to be efficacious on the basis of data from nonexperimental studies, but it is uncertain whether the measured efficacy is "far beyond what could reasonably be attributed to possible biases." Gauging the adequacy of data from these studies is very much a subjective process. There are situations in which some persons are "certain" of a therapy's efficacy while others, reviewing the same evidence, are not. This author's subjective recommendation is to insist on a very strong demonstration of efficacy in a nonexperimental study before concluding that a randomized controlled trial of the treatment in question is inappropriate. There have been too many examples (for several, see pp. 78) in which we know we would have been led astray had a controlled trial not been done. It is true, if a controlled trial is carried out and it "only" confirms the results of prior nonexperimental studies, that the patients enrolled in the trial who were not given the therapy under study would not have benefited as they might have in the absence of the trial. But if the controlled trial is not done and the therapy truly is not efficacious, then a very much larger number of patients will undergo the treatment for no good reason. Indeed, the therapy may actually be detrimental, in which case that very much larger number of patients will be harmed for lack of a controlled trial capable of determining this.

Example. During the 1960s in the United States, several drugs were being prescribed to patients who had sustained a myocardial infarction, in an effort to decrease the likelihood of reinfarction. The evidence supporting the efficacy of these drugs (estrogens, dextrothyroxine, clofibrate, and nicotinic acid) was largely or exclusively nonexperimental. A group of investigators judged this evidence to be less than definitive, and they mounted a large experimental study— the Coronary Drug Project—to more thoroughly evaluate whether the use of one of these drugs could truly reduce the rate of reinfarction.

The results of this study were disappointing, to put it mildly. Relative to the subjects given a placebo, those given clofibrate or nicotinic acid experienced no reduction in mortality from coronary disease, and those given estrogens or dextrothyroxine actually experienced an increase (Coronary Drug Project Research Group, 1970, 1972, 1973, 1975). In the United States, the use of these drugs among patients in the postinfarction period declined precipitously following the publication of these results (Friedman et al., 1983).

WHICH TYPE OF NONEXPERIMENTAL DESIGN TO CHOOSE?

Given that you are going to try to measure the efficacy of a therapy without the benefit of an experimental study, which nonexperimental approach—follow-up or case-control—is preferable? The intuitive choice, one that works well in many situations, is the follow-up approach: Patients treated in different ways are monitored and compared with respect to the rate of disease progression/complications. However, if (a) a relatively small fraction (less than 10% or so) of patients develops the progression/complications, (b) it is necessary to obtain a considerable amount of information on each study subject (e.g., related to the assessment of disease severity) and (c) if the use of the therapy itself is not too uncommon among patients with the condition, it may prove far more economical to do a case-control study. This would involve identifying persons in whom the progression/complications occurred and a sample of patients in whom these did not occur. The treatment given to members of each of the two groups would be ascertained, along with characteristics known to influence the rate of progression/complications. The greater the degree to which "cases" (i.e., patients who develop progression/complications) have received a therapeutic measure less often than controls, the greater the efficacy of that measure (see Chapter 6 for more on the analysis of and inferences from case-control studies).

Example. The study that evaluated lidocaine prophylaxis used a case-control design (Horwitz and Feinstein, 1981). For patients who died during hospitalization following an acute myocardial infarction, medical records were reviewed to determine if lidocaine had been administered and which risk factors for cardiac death were present. The investigators chose a case-control approach because these fatalities made up only about 10% of the total number of patients with myocardial infarction, and because of the time required to extract therapeutic and prognostic data from the chart of each subject. The same review was done for a sample of patients who survived their myocardial infarction, approximately equal in size to the sample of patients who died. They were chosen so as to be comparable in demographic and prognostic characteristics, but were otherwise chosen at random. The results were as follows:

Lidocaine prophylaxis	Deaths from ventricular arrhythmia ($n = 35$)*	Controls ($n = 136$)
Yes	14%	35%
No	86%	65%
Total	100%	100%

(*Deaths due to other causes excluded.)

Because a significantly ($P = 0.02$) lower proportion of cases than of controls had been given lidocaine, the data suggest that lidocaine prophylaxis is efficacious in reducing post-myocardial infarction mortality from ventricular arrhythmia.

QUESTIONS, CHAPTER 5

5-1. In the mid-1970s, concern over the safety of pertussis vaccine led a number of British physicians and parents to use diphteria/tetanus (DT) vaccine instead of the traditional diphtheria/pertussis/tetanus (DPT) vaccine. During January 1978 to June 1980, pertussis cases were identified in 21 English "health areas" and the pertussis rate was calculated as a function of type of vaccine received (Pollock et al., 1982). The results were as follows: 2,261 cases of pertussis in 250,163 children vaccinated with DPT, and 9,515 cases of pertussis in 187,595 children vaccinated with DT.

    a. What was the incidence of pertussis during this 2.5-year period in the group that received DPT vaccine? In the group that received DT vaccine?

    b. Does it seem likely that the disparity between these rates could be attributed to differences in the characteristics of the children who received the two vaccines?

5-2. You are a gynecologist at a large medical center and you would like to evaluate your success in treating ovarian cancer. You have data for patients from two periods, 1955 to 1960 and 1975 to 1980, and you wish to determine whether patient survival has improved over the two-decades interval. Therapy for ovarian cancer has changed considerably during the interval, with radiation therapy and promising chemotherapeutic agents being used to a larger extent in 1975–80. Procedures to evaluate the patients were similar between the two periods, except that lymphangiography and peritoneoscopy, techniques designed to detect the spread of ovarian cancer, were not available in 1955–60; they were used uniformly during 1975–80.

Because you are aware of the relationship between histologic type and survival, you obtain survival data specific for histologic type. Below are the (hypothetical) data for serous cystadenocarcinomas alone:

Stage (when first treated at the medical center)	1955–60		1975–80	
	% survival*	No. of subjects	% survival*	No. of subjects
Stage I (spread limited to ovaries)	60	30	70	20
Stage II (spread limited to pelvic structures)	40	50	50	40
Stages III, IV (spread beyond pelvic structures)	0	20	10	40

(*At 5 years after first treatment in the medical center.)

a. For women with serous cystadenocarcinoma treated in each time period, what is the 5-year survival (i) Adjusted for stage at diagnosis? (Use the stage distribution of all 200 patients as a standard. See Appendix, pp. 136–137, for instructions as to how to perform the adjustment.) (ii) Not adjusted for stage at diagnosis?

b. Why does the size of the difference in 5-year survival between the two time periods depend on whether or not adjustment was performed?

c. What assumptions are needed in order to decide which of the two sets of rates, adjusted or unadjusted, offers a more valid portrait of the true difference in survival from ovarian cancer (serous cystadenocarcinoma) between the two time periods?

ANSWERS

5-1. a. The cumulative incidence of pertussis in the DPT-vaccinated group was 2,261/250,163 = 903.8 per 100,000, and in the DT-vaccinated group, 9,515/187,595 = 5,072.1 per 100,000.

b. There was a greater than fivefold difference in the incidence of pertussis between the two groups of children. To judge whether the difference might have been due to something other than the effect of the vaccine, it is necessary to consider the other factors that bear on the incidence of pertussis and to what extent they may differ between the DPT- and DT-vaccinated groups. "Host" factors appear to be relatively unimportant in pertussis—most nonimmunized persons exposed to the pathogen develop the disease. In any event, it is hard to imagine how the reasons for choosing DT over DPT vaccine, reasons relating to physician and/or parental concern over possible adverse effects, could relate in an important way to a child's underlying risk of pertussis. Thus, it would seem safe to conclude from this nonexperimental study that most, if not all, of the difference in pertussis incidence between DPT- and DT-vaccinated groups was due to the use of the pertussis vaccine.

5-2. a(i). Stage-adjusted survival
Standard "weights," combined distribution:

Stage	Weight
I	(30 + 20)/200 = 0.25
II	(50 + 40)/200 = 0.45
III	(20 + 40)/200 = 0.30

Adjusted survival:

Stage	1955–60	1975–80
I	60% × 0.25 = 15.0	70% × 0.25 = 17.5
II	40% × 0.45 = 18.0	50% × 0.45 = 22.5
III, IV	0% × 0.30 = 0	10% × 0.30 = 3.0
Total, adjusted	33.0%	43.0%

a(ii).   Unadjusted (crude) survival:

Stage	1955–60	1975–80
I	60% × 0.30 = 18.0	70% × 0.20 = 14.0
II	40% × 0.50 = 20.0	50% × 0.40 = 20.0
III, IV	0% × 0.20 = 0	10% × 0.40 = 4.0
Total, unadjusted	38.0%	38.0%

b.   The difference in 5-year survival between the two time periods is 0% before adjustment, and 10% after adjustment for stage. This results from the fact that the stage distribution among the cases in the two time periods was quite different, there being a higher proportion of more advanced stages during 1975–80, and the strong relationship between stage and 5-year survival. When the stage distribution is forced (via adjustment) to be the same in the two time periods, the 10% difference in stage-specific survival that favors the recent time period is reflected in the overall survival.

c.   If the difference in stage distribution between the two time periods is real, then it is essential to adjust for stage because the higher proportion of more serious cases in 1975–80 (perhaps due to changes in patterns of referral to the medical center) in an unadjusted comparison would result in bias against finding any improvement in 5-year survival over time.

But is it possible that there has been no real change in the stage distribution, that the apparent difference is due to the fact that stage has not been assessed in the same way in 1975–80 as it was 20 years earlier? Yes: Had lymphangiography and peritoneoscopy been available in 1955–60, some women's tumors that were categorized as Stage I at that time would have been correctly categorized as Stages II–IV. The remaining women with "true" Stage I tumors would have had a better survival than would women in the original group that contained the miscategorized cases, since they, on the average, had less extensive disease.

And what would happen to the mean survival of women with Stage II–IV tumors once the "former" Stage I cases, now correctly classified, were included: It is likely that it would be greater as well because of the presence of women with less obvious tumor extension; overall, the group would have chance of survival than the original group of Stage II–IV cases.

Therefore, it is possible that, even with no change in the effectiveness of therapy over the two decades, a change in the way in which stage was determined could have produced an increase in the stage-specific survival (and thus the stage-adjusted survival). Without knowing to what extent the change in stage distribution was due to a true difference in the distribution of disease severity rather than to an altered way of identifying "stage" itself, no conclusion can be reached concerning improvement in the efficacy of therapy.

REFERENCES

Broome CV, Facklam RR, Fraser DW: Pneumococcal disease after pneumococcal vaccination. *N Engl J. Med* 1980; 303:549–552.

Coronary Drug Project Research Group: The Coronary Drug Project: Initial findings leading to modification of its research protocol. *JAMA* 1970; 214:1303–1313.

Coronary Drug Project Research Group: The Coronary Drug Project: Findings leading to further modifications of its protocol with respect to dextrothyroxine. *JAMA* 1972; 220:996–1008.

Coronary Drug Project Research Group: The Coronary Drug Project: Findings leading to discontinuation of the 2.5 mg/day estrogen group. *JAMA* 1973; 226:652–657.

Coronary Drug Project Research Group: Clofibrate and niacin in coronary heart disease. *JAMA* 1975; 231:360–381.

Friedman L, Wenger NK, Knatterud GL: Impact of the coronary drug project findings on clinical practice. *Controlled Clin Trials* 1983; 4:513–522.

Gehan EA, Freireich EJ: Non-randomized controls in cancer clinical trials. *N Engl J Med* 1974; 290:198–203.

Horwitz RI, Feinstein AR: Improved observational method for studying therapeutic efficacy: Suggestive evidence that lidocaine prophylaxis prevents death in acute myocardial infarction. *JAMA* 1981; 246:2455–2459.

Johnson FL, Thomas ED, Clark BS, Chard RL, Hartmann JR, Storb R: A comparison of marrow transplantation with chemotherapy for children with acute lymphoblastic leukemia in second or subsequent remission. *N Engl J Med* 1981; 305:846–851.

Kotzin BL, Strober S, Engleman EG, Calin A, Hoppe RT, Kansas GS, Terrell CP, Kaplan HS: Treatment of intractable rheumatoid arthritis with total lymphoid irradiation. *N Engl J Med* 1981; 305:969–975.

Levin ML, Tockman MS, Frost JK, Ball WC: Lung cancer mortality in males screened by chest x-ray and cytologic sputum examination: A preliminary report. *Cancer Res* 1982; 82:138–146.

Lindsay R, Aitken JM, Anderson JB, Hart DM, MacDonald EB, Clarke AC: Long-term prevention of postmenopausal osteoporosis by estrogen: Evidence for an increased bone mass after delayed onset of estrogen treatment. *Lancet* 1976; 1:1038–1040.

Lindsay R, MacLean A, Kraszewski A, Hart DM, Clark AC, Garwood J: Bone response to termination of oestrogen treatment. *Lancet* 1978; 1:1325–1327.

Monson RR, MacMahon B, Austin JH: Postoperative irradiation in carcinoma of the endometrium. *Cancer* 1973; 31:630–632.

Mossey JM, Shapiro E: Self-rated health: A predictor of mortality among the elderly. *Am J Public Health* 1982; 72:800–808.

Paganini-Hill A, Ross RK, Gerkins VR, Henderson BE, Arthur M, Mack TM: Menopausal estrogen therapy and hip fractures. *Ann Intern Med* 1981; 95:28–31.

Pollock TM, Miller E, Lobb J. Smith G: Efficacy of pertussis vaccination in England. *Br Med J* 1982; 285:357–359.

Sacks H, Chalmers TC, Smith H: Randomized versus historical controls for clinical trials. *Am J Med* 1982; 72:233–239.

Tovey LAD, Townley A, Stevenson BJ, Taverner J: The Yorkshire antenatal anti-D immunoglobulin trial in primigravadae. *Lancet* 1983; 2:244–246.

Van der Linden W. Pitfalls in randomized surgical trials. *Surgery* 1980; 87:258–262.

Veterans Administration Cooperative Urological Research Group: Treatment and survival of patients with cancer of the prostate. Surg Gynecol Obstet 1967; 124:1011–1017.

Vollmer WM, Wahl PW, Blagg CR: Survival with dialysis and transplantation inpatients with end-stage renal disease. *N Engl J Med* 1983; 308:1553–1558.

Weiss NS: Inferring causal relationships: Elaboration of the criterion of "dose-response." *Am J Epidemiol* 1981; 113:487–490.

Weiss NS, Ure CL, Ballard JH, Williams AR, Daling JR: Decreased risk of fractures of the hip and lower forearm with postmenopausal use of estrogen. *N Engl J Med* 1980; 303:1195–1198.

6 Therapeutic Safety

ROLE OF EXPERIMENTAL STUDIES

We have seen the heavy reliance that is placed on results of experimental studies (randomized controlled trials) in evaluating the efficacy of a given therapy. Unfortunately, experimental studies cannot contribute as much to our understanding of the adverse effects associated with these same therapies.

Experimental studies are based on samples of several dozen to, at most, several thousand subjects. Some adverse effects that bear heavily on a therapy's risk/benefit ratio are relatively uncommon and so may not occur in any one study. Even if some adverse effects are seen in the study subjects, the frequency may be too low to result in a "statistically significant" difference between the treated and untreated group.

Figure 6-1 relates the difference in the cumulative frequency of a particular adverse effect between treatment and control groups (the groups are assumed to be of equal size) to the number of subjects needed to reliably identify its association with treatment. It is evident that small, true absolute differences in the frequencies of an adverse effect between the two groups require very large numbers of subjects to enable their statistical detection. For example, it would be necessary to have enrolled nearly 1,000 treated patients to document an adverse effect that manifests itself in 1% of them, even if the occurrence of this effect in the untreated patients were only one-tenth as great. The more common the effect in the untreated patients (e.g., the upper line in Figure 6-1), the larger must be the study to detect a difference of a given magnitude.

90

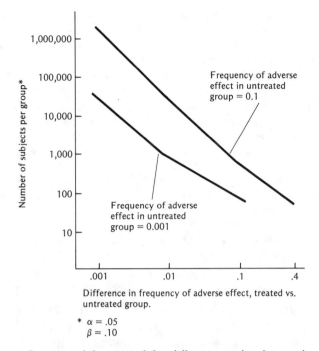

Figure 6-1. Influences of the size of the difference to be detected and the frequency of the adverse effect in the untreated group on the number of subjects needed in an experimental study.

Thus, it is no surprise that the excess risk of vaginal adenocarcinoma caused by in utero diethylstilbestrol (DES) exposure, estimated from nonexperimental data to be not more than 1 per 1,000 (Lanier et al., 1973), would not be documented in the follow-up of the daughters of the several hundred women who participated in the clinical trials of this drug (Bibbo et al., 1977; Beral and Colwell, 1981). Indeed, not a single case appeared in the latter studies.

It is instructive to review several examples of analyses of data from clinical trials that were successful in uncovering an uncommon adverse effect to get a feeling for the conditions that are needed to achieve success:

Example. Investigators at the National Cancer Institute were concerned with the possible adverse effects of alkylating agents administered in the treatment of ovarian cancer (Greene et al., 1982). From data collected in five separate clinical trials, in which a total of 1,399 subjects were enrolled, they monitored the subsequent incidence of acute leukemia. In the 998 women who received alkylating agents, 12 cases of leukemia occurred. No cases of leukemia were found in the 401 women to whom alkylating agents were not given, and only 0.11 cases would have been expected on the basis of leukemia incidence rates among women in general. This investigation was successful in documenting the high risk of leukemia because the excess risk associated with the administration of alkylating agents was indeed great, elevated by more than 100 times, and because the investigators were able to aggregate a large enough body of data so that they could virtually rule out the role of chance in producing the excess.

Example. To evaluate the role of systemic corticosteroid therapy in producing peptic ulcers, results were pooled from 71 (!) randomized controlled trials in which the occurrence of side effects was monitored (Messer et al., 1983). Fifty-five (1.8%) of 3,064 steroid-treated patients developed an ulcer, significantly more than the 0.8% of 2,897 controls. Had the data set been much smaller, this relatively small increased risk for this relatively infrequent adverse effect would have been "missed" (i.e., the incidence in the two groups would have been found to be not significantly different).[1]

The duration of use of a therapy in a clinical trial is often limited, and may be shorter than that required to produce the adverse effect. For example, retinopathy from the use of chloroquine generally develops only after 3 years of use (Bernstein, 1967). Only a very small number of clinical trials continue for more than 3 years.

Some important adverse effects may only be manifest long after drug use has been initiated. Thus, the excess incidence of vaginal adenocarcinoma in girls who were exposed in utero to DES, appearing some 15 years after exposure, could not be detected in clinical trials that evaluated the effects of DES on the immediate outcome of pregnancy.

ROLE OF NONEXPERIMENTAL STUDIES

In view of the limitations of experimental studies in the area of therapeutic safety, it is fortunate that nonexperimental studies can generally be trusted to provide more valid answers here than they can for drug efficacy. Why is this so? Because the presence of a given symptom or condition that leads to the use of a particular treatment is often unrelated to the likelihood of the patient developing the effect in question. For example, the decision to use chloroquine

---

[1]When pooling data from multiple studies, it is necessary to keep in mind the possibility that confounding may arise if both (a) the ratios of treated to untreated patients differ among the studies and (b) the frequencies with which the postulated adverse effect occurs differ among the studies. If these conditions are met, the potential distortion of the pooled results can be prevented by the "deconfounding" technique described in the Appendix (p. 136).

prophylaxis is based on considerations other than the patient's pro-
clivity to develop retinopathy, so a comparison of the frequency of
retinopathy in users and nonusers probably will be a valid one. This
contrasts with the decidedly limited validity of a nonexperimental
comparison of chloroquine users' and nonusers' rates of developing
malaria; here, it is likely that users of the drug would be those persons at highest risk of the disease, for instance, persons travelling to
or residing in areas of highest disease transmission.

Case Reports/Case Series

As a result of clinical experience with a form of therapy and/or
from reading of the experience of others, a provider of health care
develops some expectations as to the effect of that therapy. Thus,
when the health care provider perceives that an unusual effect has
occurred, he or she might take note of it and might be prompted to
look for similar effects in subsequent patients and/or report the discovery to colleagues or to an appropriate agency. This is the manner
by which many untoward effects of therapy begin to be brought to
light, whether high infection rates following certain types of surgical
procedures, anaphylaxis following administration of a drug, or, for
a more specific instance, retrolental fibroplasia following oxygen
therapy in premature infants.

Nonetheless, it is apparent that the specificity and sensitivity of
this sort of reporting system is poor. First, such reports identify far
more potential associations than would be verified if more detailed
studies could be done to corroborate the relationships. Second,
some bona fide adverse effects will not be reported as such, particularly if the incidence of the adverse effect is low, does not promptly
follow administration of therapy, or is more commonly caused by
factors other than the therapy in question. For example, more than
40 years lapsed between the time estrogens were first used in the
treatment of menopausal symptoms and the time that hypothesis-
testing studies were done to document the association of such use
with the increased incidence of endometrial cancer. Recognition
was delayed because, in part, (a) a large majority of estrogen users
did not develop endometrial cancer, (b) there was a several-year-
long interval between first use and the appearance of excess risk of
the disease, and (c) the occurrence of endometrial cancer in a postmenopausal woman is not uncommon even in the absence of exogenous estrogens.

Clearly, what is needed to evaluate therapeutic safety is the determination of the rate of the particular manifestation suspected to be an unintended effect, both in persons to whom the particular therapy is given and in those to whom it is not. The nonexperimental studies that make these comparisons are (a) cohort (follow-up) studies, which estimate the rates directly, and (b) case-control studies, which allow the estimation of relative rates.

Cohort (Follow-Up) Studies

Cohort studies first characterize persons as to whether they have received a particular therapy, and then monitor them for the occurrence of one or more symptoms, signs, or illnesses that could represent an adverse effect. The monitoring can be prospective, in persons currently being treated, or retrospective, in persons treated in the past.

An example of the *prospective* approach is the follow-up, for mortality, of patients to whom cimetidine was prescribed (Colin-Jones et al., 1983). These patients ($n = 9,928$) were identified during 1978 through British pharmacists and pharmacy records. For comparison, an age-matched sample of cimetidine nonusers was chosen from the practices of the physicians who had prescribed cimetidine. One year later, the physicians' records of both groups were reviewed to determine the patients' status. (The results and limitations of this particular comparison are described below; see example on p. 96) By way of contrast, the *retrospective* approach was employed by Walker et al. (1981) to determine if vasectomy was associated with a subsequently altered risk of myocardial infarction. During 1979 to 1980, records of the pathology department of a large prepaid health care plan were reviewed for the years 1963 to 1978 to identify men who had undergone vasectomy ($n = 4,830$). The rate of hospitalization for a first-time myocardial infarction in these men during 1972 to 1979, the years for which hospital discharge diagnoses were computerized, was compared with that of an age-matched group of male health plan members (the rates were found to be nearly identical).

The issues governing the design, conduct, and analysis of cohort studies that evaluate unintended effects of therapy are in many ways similar to those of cohort studies that evaluate other exposures (e.g., occupational, environmental, dietary). The elaboration of these issues is best left to works on epidemiology per se. Nonetheless, there are several aspects of cohort studies that call for particular emphasis.

Nature of the Comparison Group

In theory, there are two options for comparison groups. Subjects can be drawn from a population that has the condition for which the treatment is given but that has not been treated or has been treated in a different manner. Or, the comparison group can be drawn from the population of untreated persons in general, irrespective of whether they have the condition that leads to the particular therapy. What considerations guide the choice between these alternatives?

Ideally, the *comparison group should consist of untreated persons whose underlying risk (i.e., risk in the absence of the therapy) of the symptom/ sign/illness being investigated as a possible adverse effect is the same as that of the group that receives the therapy.* Persons who have the same condition as those being treated, but who themselves receive different (or no) therapy, would seem to correspond most closely to the ideal, for then any associations found cannot be ascribed to the condition itself. For example, a greatly increased risk of acute leukemia was observed in cohort studies of alkylating agent therapy for ovarian cancer (Reimer et al., 1977) and of "intensive chemotherapy" (nitrogen mustard, procarbazine, prednisone, and either vincristine or vinblastine) for Hodgkin's disease (Boivin and Hutchison, 1981). In both studies, the increase was apparent relative not only to incidence rates in the population as a whole but to rates in patients with these neoplasms who did not receive the therapies. Thus, one could rule out the possibility that the excess risk of leukemia was due solely to a predisposition to leukemia among persons with ovarian cancer or Hodgkin's disease.

There are many situations in which there is no ill-but-untreated group readily available for comparison. For example, in attempting to evaluate the long-term toxicity of DES exposure during pregnancy, it may prove impossible to find a cohort of women who were pregnant during the 1950s, were not given the drug, and who had the same indication for use (e.g., threatened spontaneous abortion) as did the DES-exposed group. Similarly, to evaluate the influence of neuroleptic agents on the incidence of breast cancer (these drugs stimulate prolactin secretion, which, in rodents, plays an etiologic role in mammary cancer), one would be hard pressed to identify women with comparable psychologic impairment to whom these agents were not given.

Remembering the guideline for selection of an appropriate comparison group, the use of persons who do not have the illness for which treatment was instituted will provide a valid result if the illness per se is not associated with the occurrence of the adverse effect. Fortunately, this is usually the case. For example, apart from its necessitating the use of penicillin, pneumococcal pneumonia is unrelated to anaphylaxis or to the development of other allergic manifestations. Thus, a valid measure of the role of penicillin in producing these allergic manifestations could be obtained by comparing their incidence in persons given penicillin with that in persons not given penicillin, irrespective of the pneumonia status of the latter group. In the same way, potential miscarriage or other reasons for prescribing DES during pregnancy probably are not themselves related to the development of vaginal adenosis in female offspring. Thus, the daughters of women who did not take DES, whether or not the women were at risk of spontaneous abortion during pregnancy, are an appropriate group for comparison with daughters of DES-exposed women when evaluating vaginal adenosis and other possible adverse effects.

Nonetheless, there will be some situations in which the lack of an ill but un-treated group for comparison will render the results of the study uninterpretable, that is, it will prove impossible to separate the influence of the therapy in producing the suspected adverse effect from the influence of the illness for which the therapy was given:

Example. In the study mentioned previously, mortality among cimetidine users was compared with that among other (nonuser) patients in general, not specifically with mortality in persons with gastric acid–related disease who did not use cimetidine (Colin-Jones et al., 1983). This choice led to some ambiguity when the investigators attempted to interpret the results of the study:

Cause of death	Cumulative mortality (per 10,000) in first follow-up year*:	
	Cimetidine user	Nonuser
All	377.7	211.7
Malignant neoplasm*		
Esophagus	7.1	1.1
Stomach	31.2	3.2
Bronchus and lung	18.1	11.8

(*Patients who died of a cancer that was diagnosed prior to initiation of cimetidine therapy excluded.)

Certainly, part of the cimetidine users' excess mortality from all causes combined was due to conditions and their complications that necessitated therapy for relief of symptoms of peptic disease, for example, gastric cancer, lymphoma, chronic liver disease. Nonetheless, even after these known antecedent conditions are excluded from the analysis, a large excess mortality for certain diseases (e.g., cancers of the esophagus, stomach, and lung) remains. While these deaths could have been due to an effect of cimetidine, it is far more likely that they were the result of a not yet diagnosed disease process that led to the use of the drug. In the absence of a comparison group with symptoms similar to those of the patients given cimetidine, it is virtually impossible to discern any true effect of this drug on short-term mortality.

Ascertainment of the Effect(s) Under Study

Whatever the group used for comparison, the recognition of a manifestation that could represent an adverse effect should be made equally well whether or not a patient has received the therapy under study. There are two ways of attempting to achieve such equal recognition: (a) ascertainment with knowledge of exposure status withheld and (b) enumeration of unambiguous criteria for the presence of the effect to be applied uniformly in treated and untreated individuals. The first of these, "blind" ascertainment, is rarely employed in nonexperimental studies of therapeutic safety because nearly always such studies must rely on physicians to document or diagnose the effect in their patients. Thus, even if the investigator assembles the data without knowledge of treatment status, the data he or she is assembling may incorporate a "detection" bias on the part of the patients' physicians.

Thus, more commonly, cohort studies attempt to equalize ascertainment using the second approach, standard criteria. While this may be difficult or impossible for potential adverse effects that often go undetected or unrecorded, (e.g., thrombophlebitis, gynecomastia), in many instances standard criteria are easily applied and pose little or no problems in interpretation, even when the standards are not very rigorous. For example, 17 cases of non-Hodgkin's lymphoma were detected among 6,297 recipients of renal transplants identified through an international transplant registry, whereas only 0.5 cases would have been expected on the basis of incidence rates in the general population (Hoover and Fraumeni, 1973). No attempt was made to standardize the criteria used to determine the presence of non-Hodgkin's lymphoma: the registry covered patients in 30 countries. Still, the association is almost certainly a real one, in part because of its magnitude, but also because of the relatively similar criteria that would have been used between these patients and the comparison populations for the diagnosis of non-Hodgkin's lymphoma. (The issue of ascertainment in the follow-up for neoplasia in renal transplant recipients is, of course, distinct from the issue discussed earlier, that is, the separation of the influence of the transplant and its associated therapy from the influence of the underlying renal disease. Studies directed at distinguishing between these possibilities—cohort studies of persons with renal failure who did not receive a transplant—are not in full agreement, but it seems clear that whatever excess risk of non-Hodgkin's lymphoma might be present in such patients is considerably smaller than what exists in the transplant recipients.)

It is important to recognize those situations in which the use of strict criteria for effect is necessary in order for the study to have validity:

> *Example.* In late 1978, investigators in the Ohio Department of Health tried to quantify the association between vaccination against A/New Jersey influenza virus (swine flu) and the occurrence of the Guillain-Barré syndrome (GBS) (Marks and Halpin, 1980). Through Health Department records they were able to enumerate the approximately 2.2 million vaccinated persons. To ascertain cases of GBS, they queried neurologists in the state for cases diagnosed during and shortly after the time the vaccination program was taking place. The investigators were concerned that there might have been selective over-ascertainment of GBS patients who had been vaccinated, since (a) the diagnosis of GBS is not always clear-cut and (b) the ascertainment of cases took place during a period in which there was considerable public speculation as to the presence of a swine flu–GBS link. Such speculation conceivably could have influenced neurologists to take account of vaccination status when considering a diagnosis of GBS. Thus, the investigators required that, in order for a case to be accepted into the study, there must have been evidence of lower-motor neuron weakness of acute onset. Patients given a diagnosis of GBS without such weakness were excluded. (In addition, vaccinated and nonvaccinated cases were compared in terms of severity—if a diagnostic bias were present, the vaccinated cases would be expected to have been less severe on average—and no difference was found.)

Cohort Studies as a Means of Surveillance for Adverse Effects

An important function of cohort studies of therapeutic safety is hypothesis generation, the systematic appraisal of therapies for clues to unsuspected adverse effects. For the generation of clues, we ask for less in terms of methodologic rigor than when testing specified hypotheses but more in terms of breadth of therapies and/ or possible effects being examined.

Among the systematic approaches to searching for adverse effects of drugs, there is no best one for all effects. In particular, the surveillance method that searches for relatively acute adverse reactions will differ from the one that explores late effects.

Those adverse effects that occur soon (minute to days) after administration of therapy can most easily be studied by monitoring patients during a hospital stay (Miller, 1973). All therapies are recorded and the patients' records are monitored for the occurrence of one or more of a large number of specified events (e.g., convulsions, electrocardiographic or electrolyte changes). The respective rates of each of these events in recipients and nonrecipients of various therapies are systematically compared. (Some surveillance programs of this type also obtain the judgment of the patients' physicians as to whether an adverse event is therapy-related.)

Example. Data on 1,602 medical inpatients of two Boston hospitals over a 3-year period were screened to identify drug-related causes of gastrointestinal hemorrhage that developed during hospitalization (Slone et al., 1969). The 157 patients who had received the diuretic ethacrynic acid had an unusually high frequency of this complication. Data were available on several important confounding factors (heparin use, blood urea nitrogen level, sex); after adjustment for these there was a two-to-three fold excess risk in ethacrynic acid users relative to the risk in nonusers. Two aspects of this analysis are of note: (a) Because of the hypothesis-generating nature of the study, the criterion for hemorrhage was simply a physician's notation of this condition on the patient's discharge summary. No attempt was made to standardize diagnoses of hemorrhage or of any other potential adverse effect, for this task would have been beyond the study's resources. Indeed, no attempt was made to distinguish the site(s) of bleeding in the analysis (e.g., upper vs. lower gastrointestinal tract). (b) In this study, the patients' physicians were asked to provide their opinions as to whether complications that developed during hospitalization were the result of drug administration and, if so, of which drug. None of the 32 cases of hemorrhage that occurred in ethacrynic acid users was attributed to the drug, underscoring the limitations of "case reporting" as a means of providing clues about the occurrence of adverse drug effects.

The virtue of in-hospital surveillance for adverse effects lies in its efficiency relative to other methods: Large numbers of drugs and other therapeutic measures are prescribed in hospitals, and patients can be followed with relatively little expense by means of their charts. Still, an immense number of patients must be evaluated to adequately monitor drugs that are prescribed with low frequency in such a setting or to detect adverse effects that occur with low frequency. For example, in a surveillance program conducted in 1,669 pediatric inpatients, only six drugs (apart from oxygen, vitamins, and intravenous fluids) were administered to more than 200 children (Mitchell et al., 1979). Only two effects, fever and anemia, occurred in more than 100 children, and, of course, in most instances these did not result from the use of a drug.

To uncover adverse effects that do not occur until weeks or years after therapy, the experience of recipients and nonrecipients outside the hospital setting must be monitored. The evaluation of the long-term safety of pharmaceutical agents has been particularly amenable to study. Large numbers of persons (tens to hundreds of thousands) who have had drugs prescribed to them have been identified through computerized pharmacy records in prepaid health care plans in the United States (Friedman, 1978; Jick et al., 1981) and in England through a central Pricing Authority (Skegg and Doll, 1981). Follow-up of the patients for conditions that might represent untoward drug effects over a period of several years has been accomplished through physician checklists and tumor registry data (Friedman, 1978), computerized hospital discharge diagnoses (Jick et al., 1981), or a population-based morbidity and mortality reporting system (Skegg and Doll, 1981).

It is the ability of such studies to identify large numbers of users of drugs that makes them so appealing for generating hypotheses. For example, in the study of Friedman (1978) and of Friedman and Ury (1980), among 143,574 users of at least one drug there were 16,072 users of belladonna alkaloids, 4,867 users of indomethacin, and 5,834 users of phenobarbital. However, there is a price to be paid for these numbers, and it is in the quality of the data.

First, often it is unclear, without obtaining additional information, whether the drug use in fact preceded the development of the condition being evaluated as a possible adverse effect. This ambiguity can arise because the data systems have no means of ensuring that the symptoms/signs/illnesses that are recorded are only those that are new, and, if the ascertainment of illness is through review of hospital records (as is often the case), drugs used prior to the first hospital discharge diagnosis may have been part of outpatient therapy for the illness or have been for the symptoms it produced prior to diagnosis, and thus the drugs would have no etiologic significance.

Example. In the study of Skegg and Doll (1981), strong associations were found between kaolin (a constituent of antidiarrheal preparations) and rectal cancer, and between the anticonvulsant phenytoin and brain tumors. As the authors point out, almost certainly neither association represented an adverse drug effect, but rather the use of the drug for early symptoms of the underlying malignancy.

Second, the ascertainment of the symptoms/signs/illnesses is usually not standardized in any way, since it is based on medical records. An attempt to augment this ascertainment with diagnosis checklists completed by physicians met with limited success (Friedman, 1978). For example, a comparison of these checklists with the outpatient medical records of 300 patients taking the antibiotic clindamycin revealed substantial underreporting on the checklists: Only 2 of 10 patients who developed diarrhea during the 8-week period following antibiotic use would have been detected.

Finally, apparent drug–disease associations may be due to the action of one or more of the many unmeasured factors in these studies that predispose patients both to drug use and to the suspected effect. The association between dioctyl sodium sulfosuccinate, a fecal softening agent, and chronic skin ulcers found in the study of Skegg and Doll (1981) was attributed by the investigators to the mutual association of constipation and ulcers to a third factor, physical immobility.

Case-Control Studies

A case-control study evaluating therapeutic safety starts by identifying persons who have developed a particular symptom, sign, or illness "cases". It then identifies persons without the symptom/sign/illness ("controls") who are otherwise comparable with the cases, and in both groups ascertains the proportion in which the therapy under investigation has been received. To the extent that this proportion is increased among cases relative to controls, there is support for the contention that the symptom/sign/illness represents an adverse effect of the therapy.

Are Case-Control Studies Really Necessary?

To many nonepidemiologists there is something unaesthetic about case-control studies. After all, why look for possible adverse effects in this backwards sort of way? The answer is that for some adverse effects—those that are uncommon even in persons who received the therapies that produced them—there are no alternative means of identifying them. And, even though rare, some adverse effects are serious enough that knowledge of their presence can have a strong bearing on the decision to administer the therapy in question.

Earlier in this chapter we saw that randomized trials of DES during pregnancy failed to uncover the association with vaginal adenocarcinoma in the female children: Even after several hundred of the girls born to women who participated in these studies were located and examined 15 to 20 years later, no cases were found in either the DES-exposed or the comparison group (Bibbo et al., 1977; Beral and Colwell, 1981). These negative results can be attributed to the fact that vaginal adenocarcinoma is a rare enough condition, even in DES-exposed girls, that a true association with DES exposure could be missed in a group of this size. The same problem can plague a cohort study. For example, Lanier et al. (1973) monitored the incidence of cancer through the teenage years in 804 DES-exposed girls and also failed to find a case of vaginal adenocarcinoma.

It was through case-control studies that the association between in utero DES exposure and vaginal adenocarcinoma was identified. In the first study of this subject, for example, 7 of 8 cases had been exposed to DES, whereas fewer than 1 of 8 would have been expected on the basis of the frequency in controls (Herbst et al., 1971). It was largely on the basis of these data, and those documenting the severity of this cancer, that the Food and Drug Administration withdrew approval for the use of DES during pregnancy. This action was taken despite the fact that only a very small fraction of DES-exposed girls will suffer this adverse effect.

Obtaining a Valid Case-Control Comparison

In a case-control study that evaluates the safety of therapy, the function of a control group is as follows: to estimate the frequency with which a particular therapy would have been administered to persons who have developed the suspected adverse effect if the therapy itself played no causal role. Thus, an ideal control group is one that consists of individuals (a) who are identical to the cases with respect to the distribution of all characteristics that influence the likelihood of receiving the therapy *and* that, independent of their relation to the likelihood of receiving the therapy, are also related to the occurrence of the symptom/sign/illness under study or to its recognition, and (b) in whom a history of having received the therapy can be measured in a manner that is identical in accuracy to that used for cases.

There is no one way of defining controls that is best for every study. The choice is influenced largely by (a) the source from which the cases have been identified, (b) the influence of the treatment on the tendency to diagnose the suspected adverse effect, (c) the relationship of the condition(s) for which the therapy is administred to the occurrence of this effect, and (d) the kind of information on treatment history that can be obtained.

Source of cases: Population-based or not? When an investigator is able to identify all cases arising from a defined group of individuals, he or she generally chooses as controls a sample from other members of the defined group who have not developed the symptom/sign/illness.[2] For example, three studies that explored the possibility that postmenopausal estrogens might alter a user's risk of breast cancer (Ross et al., 1980; Hoover et al., 1981; Brinton et al., 1981) identified cases within defined populations: members of a prepaid health care plan, residents of a retirement community, and enrollees for longitudinal monitoring at cancer detection clinics. Controls were, respectively, a sample of other women in the health care plan, other residents of the retirement community, and other women undergoing screening. This choice allowed some degree of comparability among cases and controls with respect to a wide range of demographic characteristics (e.g., age, socioeconomic status) that relate both to estrogen use and to incidence of breast cancer. Also, this comparability could be achieved without having to sacrifice comparability of ascertainment of prior estrogen use (see below).

In many instances, however, the cases available for study do not relate to any defined population. Commonly, cases are chosen from persons who have selected a certain provider and/or institution for their care. In such instances, it is usually valid (and convenient) to

[2]Strictly speaking, to enable the control group's experience to provide the most accurate estimate of the frequency with which of therapy has been administered in that population, persons who develop the symptom/sign/illness should be included as "controls" in proportion to their numbers in that population (Greenland and Thomas, 1982). This refinement, while appropriate, is seldom implemented. Its omission introduces virtually no bias until a high proportion of treated individuals develops the adverse effect (say, more than 20%. In such a situation, it is likely that a follow-up study would be done instead).

select controls who are similar to the cases with respect to choice of health care provider/institution, excluding those who have conditions believed to be related to the treatment under study. So, when Kelsey et al. (1981) examined the possibility of an estrogen–breast cancer relationship by studying cancer cases from three Connecticut hospitals, controls were chosen from those admitted to inpatient surgical services at those same hospitals. Excluded as potential controls, however, were women on the gynecology service, as it was felt that a number of them would have conditions that resulted from estrogen use (e.g., endometrial hyperplasia and carcinoma). The hope was that the remainder of the women admitted for surgery reflected closely the patterns of estrogen use in a hypothetical population whose members, if they were to have developed breast cancer, would have sought care in one of the three study hospitals.

What can be learned from studies that select as cases only those patients who have received the therapy in question? The British Committee on Safety of Medicines based a study on the reports they received of women who sustained a cardiovascular "event" who had been using oral contraceptives. In another study, in the United States, an attempt was made to identify users of oral contraceptives who developed endometrial cancer prior to 40 years of age. Both studies have produced important data on the safety of oral contraceptives, but only because there was heterogeneity within the type of therapy (i.e., oral contraceptives of different formulations) and because there were some data external to the study to help gauge the way in which the heterogeneity would have been expected to manifest itself (i.e., some data on the relative frequency of use of the various oral contraceptive preparations). Thus, when Meade et al. (1980) analyzed the type of oral contraceptive used by the British women reported as having sustained a cardiovascular event, they found an overrepresentation of preparations with high progestogen levels relative to that expected on the basis of sales by British retail pharmacists. In the American women who had taken oral contraceptives and who developed endometrial cancer, 19 of 30 had taken Oracon (Silverberg et al., 1977), a far higher proportion than would have been anticipated on the basis of Oracon's share of the U.S. oral contraceptive market.

It must be remembered that these studies of heterogeneity among treated persons provide evidence only of the *relative* safety of one preparation vis-à-vis another. For example, Oracon users could be overrepresented among endometrial cancer patients who used oral contraceptives because either Oracon predisposes the user to the disease or the use of other preparations reduces the indicence of the disease. The only way to distinguish between these possibilities is to do the more conventional type of case-control study in which women with and without the cancer (selected without regard to the use of the pill) are compared regarding their prior use of oral contraceptives. Indeed, when this was done, both an excess of Oracon use and a deficit of use of other oral contraceptives was found in women with endometrial cancer (Weiss and Sayvetz, 1980)

Influence of treatment on detection of the suspected adverse effect The recognition by physicians of signs, symptoms, and illnesses is imperfect, and sometimes it is influenced by the patients' previous therapy history. For instance, it has been suggested that physicians are more likely to perform diagnostic tests for endometrial cancer in women using estrogens than in other women (Horwitz and Feinstein, 1978). If this is true, and if some cases of endometrial cancer never become sufficiently symptomatic to elicit diagnostic activity, then a spurious (or spuriously large) estrogen–endometrial cancer association could arise.

The same sort of bias might be present when trying to determine if estrogen use predisposes patients to gallstone disease. Many women who have gallstones never have them diagnosed (Gracie and Ransohoff, 1982). Compared with such women, those in whom the diagnosis is made might be expected, on the average, to see a physician on a regular basis and to seek active medical intervention (e.g., diagnostic testing and surgery) for symptoms. These are also characteristics that, on the average, estrogen users might be expected to have to a greater extent than nonusers. Thus, if estrogen-use histories were compared between women diagnosed with (or treated surgically for) gallstones and a "typical" control group, falsely large estimates of an association could be obtained.

Concerns such as these led one group of investigators, when conducting a case-control study of endometrial cancer, to pick a control group that underwent the same degree of diagnostic evaluation as did the cases; they chose women without endometrial cancer who underwent uterine dilatation and currettage (D&C) or endometrial biopsy (Horwitz and Feinstein, 1978). Their results, in contrast to those of nearly all other studies of the subject (in which controls were not required to have undergone these diagnostic tests), showed virtually no association between estrogen use and endometrial cancer; there were nearly identical patterns of estrogen use in cases and controls. Unfortunately, in the process of eliminating one source of bias (that relating to differential cancer detection in users and nonusers), their design created another: Those postmenopausal women who undergo a D&C or endometrial biopsy but who do not have endometrial cancer generally have a bleeding disorder caused by a hyperplastic process in the endometrium. A common cause of endometrial hyperplasia is estrogen use, and so a history of estrogen use among such women would be very common. Using them as controls could (and did) nullify any true association of endometrial cancer with estrogen use.

Despite the fact that this strategy (of choosing controls from patients undergoing the diagnostic test(s) for the suspected adverse effect) did not "work" for endometrial cancer, there probably are some situations in which its use has merit. One might be the study of a possible estrogen–gallstone disease association, for there is no reason to believe that an association exists between estrogen use and the presence of symptoms that lead to a negative cholecystogram or ultrasound test.

One other, often-expressed concern when controls are chosen from persons who have not been evaluated for the suspected adverse effect is as follows: To the extent that there are cases mixed into this group, will not the resulting contamination lead to the case and control groups being artificially similar with respect to a history of having received the therapy? Such concern will be unwarranted any time the prevalence of the suspected adverse effect is low (which is most of the time), for the inclusion of an occasional occult case in a large group of noncases will have only a small impact on the results.

Influence of the condition for which the therapy is administered on the occurrence of the symptom/sign/illness   Controls should be matched to cases with regard to indication for treatment only if the indication itself is a risk factor for the symptom/sign/illness that defines the case group. Such matching is not often needed—rarely are both the condition being treated and the treatment given under suspicion as possibly causing an adverse effect. Nonetheless, there are instances in which failure to match (or otherwise control) for "indication" leads to an ambiguous result. For example, the use of "minor" tranquilizers among persons injured in vehicular accidents was compared with that among persons chosen at random from the population (Skegg et al., 1979). During the 3-month period preceding an accident, cases were five times more likely than controls to have been prescribed one of these agents. While this result could indicate an adverse effect of minor tranquilizers, it could as well be interpreted to indicate an underlying tendency for persons to whom these drugs are prescribed to have vehicular accidents. Since the investigators were unable to match on, and had no data available to control for, the "need" for these tranquilizers, both interpretations remain viable.

The kind of information on treatment history that can be obtained No matter how comparable a control and a case are in other respects, differences between them in the ability to ascertain a history of therapy will distort the results of a study, and possibly invalidate it altogether. Ideally, then, such ascertainment should be identical for cases and controls, with no opportunity for bias based on awareness of subsequent events. This ideal is met occasionally, most often when treatment records compiled prior to the occurrence of the suspected adverse effects are available. For example, in the study of breast cancer by Hoover et al. (1981), outpatient records of women prior to their diagnosis (and prior to a corresponding date for controls) were reviewed for possible hormone and other drug exposures. This review was done without knowledge of the case/control status of the women whose records were being reviewed.

However, in most case-control studies of therapeutic safety, it is necessary to rely on the memory of the subject. Records of therapy, particularly drug therapy, are usually not easy to assemble, and indeed may not be available. (The breast cancer study that did review records was conducted in a prepaid health care plan in which both the necessary inpatient and outpatient data were available for each subject.) For many forms of therapy, particularly surgical procedures or drugs taken for extended periods of time, memory can be trusted to be both sensitive and specific. For instance, women's statements of prior hysterectomy/oophorectomy and long-term menopausal estrogen use have been evaluated against medical records and found to be quite accurate (Jick et al., 1980; Brinton et al., 1981).

As might be expected, a subject's memory will be not so accurate for short-term drug therapy, particularly if it occurred in the not so recent past. Yet some of these short-term exposures could be associated with adverse effects. Drug therapy of even a few days' duration in pregnancy, for example (particularly in the first trimester), could be associated with abnormalities in the children. Yet the ability of mothers of abnormal and normal newborns to remember events of early pregnancy may vary considerably, and data from comparisons of two groups such as these must be interpreted with some caution. One approach to minimizing this type of recall bias has been to compare drugs taken by mothers of children with a particular type of abnormality (or collection of related abnormalities) with those taken by mothers of children with all *other* abnormalities. Presumably, the recall by women in the two groups would be comparable. Unless the drug were associated with a large number of different abnormalities, such a comparison should offer a relatively unbiased evaluation of the drug's safety.

> *Example.* In a case-control study of birth defects, women who had just delivered a child in one of several hospitals were interviewed (Rosenberg et al., 1983). The use of diazepam during the first trimester of pregnancy was equally common in mothers of children with isolated cleft palate or cleft lip (with or without cleft palate) as in the combined group of mothers of children with any other malformation. Thus, assuming that diazepam does not produce a broad range of birth defects, the development of oral clefts during fetal life does not appear to be related to exposure to this drug.

Incorporating Results of Case-Control Studies into the Decision-Making Process

When trying to arrive at a decision regarding the use of a therapy, it is necessary to balance rates (and severity) of any adverse effects against rates (and severity) of progression/complications of the condition for which the therapy is administered. So, even if it is conceded that case-control studies are capable of identifying the *existence* of an adverse effect, the important question of its *frequency* following treatment is left unresolved.

Fortunately, once a case-control study has indicated an association of therapy with an unintended effect and the effect is judged to be a result of therapy, it is usually possible to derive a reasonable estimate of the frequency with which the effect occurs. This estimate is obtained in two steps. First, it is necessary to calculate the incidence of the unintended effect in persons given the treatment in question relative to that in other persons. While the case-control study measures only the frequency with which the *treatment* has been administered, the relative incidence of the adverse *effect* can be approximated as illustrated in Table 6-1. In the example, the data indicate a greater frequency of oral contraceptive use among young women with myocardial infarction than among controls, the incidence in users being 2.8 times that in nonusers.

Table 6-1. Method of Estimating Relative Incidence of an Adverse Effect

General	Unintended effect: Present	Unintended effect: Absent	*Example*	Myocardial infarction[a]: Yes	Myocardial infarction[a]: No
Therapy administered — Yes	a	b	Current oral contraceptive use: — Yes	21	17
Therapy administered — No	c	d	Current oral contraceptive use: — No	26	59
	a + c	b + d		47	76

$$\text{Relative incidence} = \frac{a/c}{b/d} = \frac{a \times d}{b \times c} \qquad \text{Relative incidence} = \frac{21 \times 59}{26 \times 17} = 2.8$$

[a]Deaths in women aged 30 to 39 years (Mann and Inman, 1975).

The explanation as to why these frequencies of "exposure" can be manipulated to produce an estimate of relative incidence (often termed "relative risk") is contained in introductory epidemiology textbooks (MacMahon and Pugh, 1970; Schlesselman, 1982), as are the assumptions required for the estimate to be a valid one (principally, a cumulative incidence of the unintended effect in exposed persons of less than 20 to 25%).

The second step in estimating the incidence of an adverse effect involves multiplying the value obtained for relative incidence by the underlying rate of the effect in persons who have not received the therapy. The underlying rate can be obtained in one of several ways, often from published rates for populations in whom the therapy has not been used or in which the large majority of cases are not related to the therapy.

> *Example.* You look up the mortality rate from myocardial infarction in 30 to 39-year-old women during a recent period, just before oral contraceptive use became widespread, and find it to be 1.9 per 100,000 per year. Thus, the annual mortality rate from this cause in an oral contraceptive user would be expected to be about $2.8 \times 1.9/100,000/\text{year} = 5.4/100,000/\text{year}$.

What if you are not quite sure of the underlying rate you have identified; what if it might not quite be the one that prevails in your particular untreated population? Simply choose a range of plausible values for the rate, and over the whole of the range calculate a rate of the unintended effect in treated persons. Incorporate each of the resulting rates, one at a time, into the weighing of risks and benefits of the therapy (e.g., through decision analysis). For most therapies, the decision to use or not use the therapy will be the same regardless of the actual rate of the adverse effect (within the plausible range).

Case-Control Studies as a Means of Surveillance for Adverse Effects

The role of case-control studies in systematically uncovering possible adverse effects of therapy is limited to studies of those relatively few conditions in which most cases are iatrogenic. For example, the occurrence of a skin rash or vomiting in a hospitalized patient is often due to a treatment. A comparison of the therapies administered to such patients with those administered to a sample of other patients can potentially identify differences that would indicate a causal connection.

In a similar way, patients with anaphylaxis, hepatic failure, or aplastic anemia—perhaps selected from hospital admission logs—could be compared with controls for drugs received shortly prior to the occurrence of the first symptoms of illness.

ASSOCIATION BETWEEN THE USE OF A THERAPY AND THE OCCURRENCE OF AN UNINTENDED EFFECT: WHEN DOES IT REPRESENT CAUSATION?

There are several possible explanations for an association between treatment and unintended effect, and only one of these is that the treatment caused the effect. First, measurement errors could be responsible: Perhaps discovery of an adverse effect was incomplete, but less so in patients who received the treatment. Second, the patient groups being evaluated for the occurrence of an unintended effect (or, in a case-control study, for a history of having received the therapy) could be dissimilar regarding their underlying risk of the effect, leading to an apparent association with therapy when none truly exists. Finally, the association could simply be due to chance: The experience of the particular sample of subjects in the study may not really reflect that of the larger group of individuals to whom the findings are to be generalized.

Now, the means of distinguishing between these possible explanations is to a large extent subjective, and thus it is by no means infallible. Indeed, we are never able to *prove* that a cause-and-effect relationship exists; we are able only to *infer* it from available evidence. Fortunately, there are some guidelines that have served well in the past.

1. Determine the degree to which the incidence of the unintended effect is increased in persons receiving the therapy relative to that in other persons. Does there appear to be an association that

cannot be explained entirely by the presence of bias in measurement and/or incomparability of treated and untreated persons? The greater the relative incidence, the less likely it is that the above non-causal explanations could account for it.

What about the P value as a measure of the "strength" of an association? The P value is calculated for another important but narrower purpose: It answers the question, "What would be the likelihood of observing this degree of excess risk (or more) if there were no true association between therapy and the effect?" In arriving at an answer, the P value takes into account not only the size of the association but the number of subjects studied. For any given difference, a study with a large number of subjects will produce a smaller P value than will one with a small number. But, of course, the number of subjects enrolled in a study is controlled primarily by practical considerations and so must not be a factor when trying to assess the presence of a biological relationship.

Let's say that 7% of controls had been given drug X during the past year. It is far easier to attribute causality if 90% of cases had received drug X during that time than if 10% had received it, even if in both instances the case-control differences had been "statistically significant" to the same degree. In clinical epidemiologic studies, there almost always are too many sources of confounding and bias to be confident that the difference between 7% and 10% reflects the causal influence of drug X in producing the effect, no matter what the P value. A difference between 7% and 90%, however, similar to that seen for DES and vaginal adenocarcinoma, is harder to account for fully by noncausal explanations.

2. The more plausible the association between therapy and effect, in terms of knowledge gained in other areas, the more we are inclined to accept the association as representing cause and effect. Thus, the results of case-control studies showing differences in the prior use of postmenopausal estrogens by women with endometrial cancer and controls were widely accepted as indicative of a causal connection, partly because the case-control differences in use were large but also because (a) prolonged exposure to elevated levels of endogenous estrogens was known to be associated with an increased risk of endometrial cancer; (b) the case-control difference was present only for "long" durations (i.e., several or more years) of use; and (c) the rates of endometrial cancer in the population rapidly rose and fell in parallel with the level of the population's consumption of estrogens. This observation made it hard to accept the alternative hypothesis for the presence of the association, that is, that

the conditions necessitating the use of estrogens (e.g., hot flashes) were risk factors for endometrial cancer even in the absence of estrogen use. It was simply implausible that the prevalence of these necessitating conditions was rising and falling over such a relatively short period of time.

3. Absolute "proof" that a therapy produces a particular unintended effect is *never* forthcoming. Causes are inferred, not observed, and inferences require subjective processes that often differ among individuals. So, while the association between estrogens and endometrial cancer has been widely judged to reflect cause and effect, there has by no means been unanimity in this regard. Yet, it is necessary to attempt to draw inferences of cause and effect, even from inevitably incomplete data, for the alternative is to make no inference at all, which would preclude taking preventive or therapeutic action.

QUESTIONS, CHAPTER 6

6-1. In December 1980, cyclosporine replaced azathioprine as the drug with which physicians at Stanford University attempted to achieve immunosuppression in their patients undergoing cardiac transplantation. They noted that in the 32 patients who received a transplant after that date and who survived for 1 year, the mean serum creatinine rose from a presurgery value of 1.3 to 2.1 mg/dl ($P <$ 0.01). Other measures of glomerular filtration rate were also depressed after transplantation. What other patient group's experience should be reviewed for comparison to determine whether the administration of cyclosporine has an adverse effect on renal function?

6-2. There has been a widely held belief among physicians that the occurrence of psychiatric disorders in general, and depression in particular, is inordinately common in women who have undergone a hysterectomy. To determine whether this association is indeed present, and to better delineate the possible causal role of the hysterectomy itself, a follow-up study was conducted (Barker, 1968). Female residents of Dundee, Scotland, who had undergone a hysterectomy during 1960 to 1964 were identified through hospital records. The large majority of these operations had been performed for nonmalignant conditions. For comparison, a sample of Dundee women who had had a cholecystectomy during the same period were identified. Records of referrals to psychiatrists in that city were examined through 1966 (i.e., a minimum of 2 years of follow-up) to locate names of women in both cohorts.

In the first 2 years after surgery, 3.2% of the hysterectomy cohort had been referred to a psychiatrist, in contrast to only 1.2% of the cholecystectomy cohort ($P < 0.01$ for the age-adjusted difference). The observed association was not attributable to the simultaneous removal of the ovaries of women in the hysterectomy group, since only 19% also had undergone oophorectomy and their rate of referral was similar to that of the hysterectomy group as a whole. Neither could the association be explained by a higher measured level of presurgical psychiatric morbidity in women undergoing hysterectomy, for prior to surgery their rate of referral had been nearly the same as that of women in the cholecystectomy group. Finally, by including women undergoing cholecystectomy for comparison, the author could exclude the possibility that surgical procedures in general were responsible for the increased psychiatric referral rate.

Nonetheless, despite the observed association and these strengths of the study design, you have an important reservation about concluding that hysterectomy predisposes patients to psychiatric morbidity. What is it?

6-3. Following the publication in the *New England Journal of Medicine* of the results of several case-control studies that examined the relationship of diazepam use during the first trimester of pregnancy to the occurrence of oral clefts in the offspring, two investigators wrote a letter to the editor (Shiono and Mills, 1984). They stated that "the problem with the [case-control] approach is that using normal controls might lead to underreporting of exposure, whereas using [other] malformed controls might result in diazepam-induced malformations in the control group. In either instance, an erroneous estimate of risk would result."

They provided data from a follow-up study that they said "avoids these pitfalls," in which the use of diazepam (and other drugs) was ascertained during an interview at the first prenatal visit.

	Oral cleft:		
	Yes	No	
First trimester exposure to diazepam: Yes	1	853	854
No	31	32,364	32,395

a. What was the risk of oral cleft in a child whose mother had used diazepam during the first trimester of pregnancy?
b. What was that risk relative to the risk in children who were not so exposed?
c. The data from the follow-up study that the investigators presented also have limitations, relative to those from case-control studies, in evaluating a potential diazepam–oral cleft association. What do you believe to be the main one?

6-4. On learning of several laboratory studies suggesting that cardiac glycosides inhibit tumor growth, two investigators decided to do a case-control study (Goldin and Safa, 1984). They reviewed the charts of 69 patients who died in their hospital; in 21 patients the cause of death was cancer. Only one of these patients had been treated previously with digitalis preparations, in contrast to 18 of 48 patients who died from other causes.

a. From these data, can you estimate the risk of death from cancer in persons who used digitalis preparations relative to the risk in other persons? If so, what is that relative risk? If not, why not?

b. What is the most likely reason that these results overstate the influence of digitalis preparations on the occurrence of death from cancer?

ANSWERS

6-1. The investigators faced the task of separating the effects of cyclosporine administration from other aspects of cardiac transplantation and its physiologic consequences as factors responsible for the deterioration in renal function. Data were available to them on patients receiving cyclosporine for another indication, renal transplantation. However, these data were of limited value, for any adverse effect on renal function of the drug could have been swamped by the other threats to renal function in such patients.

Therefore, the investigators examined renal function in a comparison cohort, cardiac transplant patients who underwent their surgery before cyclosporine therapy was instituted (i.e., before December 1980) (Myers et al., 1984). There were 47 such patients who survived at least 1 year; all had received another immunosuppressive agent, azathioprine. Their mean serum creatinine after the transplantation was, if anything, somewhat lower than it had been (1.0 vs. 1.3 mg/dl prior to surgery).

These results argue strongly that cyclosporine produces renal dysfunction, although it should not be forgotten that the following assumptions are being made: (a) that there were no other changes in the care of heart transplant patients introduced at about the same time as cyclosporine that produce renal damage and (b) that there have been no trends over time in the propensity of patients undergoing heart transplantation to develop renal damage.

6-2. The main limitation of this study lies in the insensitive nature of the measure of psychiatric morbidity (i.e., referral to a psychiatrist), and of possible bias in that measure. It is not that you believe the investigator to have been biased in ascertaining the occurrence of psychiatric referral among members of the two cohorts. Rather, you are concerned that (a) only a small percentage of women with psychiatric morbidity are referred to a psychiatrist and (b) referral of an individual patient by her physician may be prompted by his or her belief that women are prone to suffer emotionally following a hysterectomy. Far more convincing would have been a study, otherwise designed as well as this one, that in a standardized and unbiased way obtained a direct measurement of psychiatric functioning (e.g., by personal interview) in the two groups of women.

6-3. a.   Risk of oral cleft = 1/854.

b.   Relative risk = $1/854 \div 31/32364 = 1.22$.

c.   This study has eliminated both potential "pitfalls" that it cites: There is no bias in the ascertainment of diazapam use relative to oral cleft occurrence, since knowledge of the presence or absence of the malformation occurred after the drug history was obtained; and the comparison group is not restricted to children with other conditions that could have been associated with diazepam exposure.

Unfortunately, it has replaced these pitfalls with another: It has the ability to reliably identify only a very large association between diazepam use and oral clefts. For example, even if the true incidence ratio had been 3.0, this study would have had only about a 45% chance of finding a significant difference (at the 5% level) in the occurrence of oral clefts between the offspring of diazepam users and non-users. [See Appendix for the means by which this percentage (the "power" of the study) was determined.] Note than even in more than 33,000 pregnancies, only 32 babies with clefts were available for study. A case-control study, whatever its problems may or may not be in this instance with respect to accurate ascertainment of diazepam use, could very likely achieve a larger sample of such cases, with a corresponding increase in power. The rarer the suspected adverse effect, the more a case-control study will be needed if the effect is to be identified.

6-4. a. In a case-control study of death from cancer, it is possible to estimate the relative cancer mortality associated with use of a particular therapy by dividing the odds that cases have been exposed to digitalis by the odds that controls have been exposed:

	Patients with cancer	Patients dying of other causes (controls)
Used digitalis:		
Yes	1	18
No	20	20

$$\text{Relative mortality} = \frac{1/20}{18/20} = 0.06$$

If this case-control comparison were valid (it is not, see below), it would suggest that the cancer mortality of users of digitalis preparations is only 6% that of nonusers.

b. This study is flawed primarily by the nature of the comparison group. It is likely that a sizable proportion of the group chosen—persons who died of causes other than cancer—died of cardiovascular disease and thus would contain an inordinately high number of patients who had received digitalis preparations. Even if the use of digitalis among cancer patients were perfectly typical of the population as a whole (i.e., no true association), the use of this particular control group would lead to the finding of an apparent protective effect of these drugs. Indeed, when the digitalis–cancer association was investigated by means of more appropriate comparisons, a suggestion of a modest *increase* in risk was found (Friedman, 1984).

REFERENCES

Barker MG: Psychiatric illness after hysterectomy. *Br Med J* 1968; 2:91–95.

Beral V, Colwell L: Randomised trial of high doses of stilboestrol and esthisterone therapy in pregnancy: Long-term follow-up of the children, *J Epidemiol Community Health* 1981; 35:155–160.

Bernstein HN: Chloroquine ocular toxicity. *Surv Ophthalmol* 1967; 12:415–417.

Bibbo M, Gill WB, Freidoon A, Blough R, Fang VS, Rosenfield RL, Schumacher GFB, Sleeper K, Sonek MG, Wied GL: Follow-up study of male and female offspring of DES-exposed mothers. *J Obstet Gynecol* 1977; 49:1–8.

Boivin JF, Hutchison GB: Leukemia and other cancers after radiotherapy and chemotherapy for Hodgkin's disease. *JNCI* 1981; 67:751–760.

Brinton LA, Hoover RN, Szklo M, Fraumeni JF: Menopausal estrogen use and risk of breast cancer. *Cancer* 1981; 47:2517–2522.

Colin-Jones DG, Langman MJS, Lawson DH, Vessey MP: Postmarketing surveillance of the safety of cimetidine: 12 month mortality report. *B Med J* 1983; 286:1713–1716.

Friedman GD: Monitoring of drug effects in outpatients: Development of a program to detect carcinogenesis, in Ducrot H et al. (eds): *Computer Aid to Drug Therapy and to Drug Monitoring*, Amsterdam, North-Holland Publishing Company, 1978; pp. 55–62.

Friedman GD: Digitalis and breast cancer. *Lancet* 1984; 2:875.

Friedman GD, Ury HK: Initial screening for carcinogenicity of commonly used drugs. *JNCI* 1980; 65:723–733.

Goldin AG, Safa AR: Digitalis and cancer. *Lancet* 1984; 1:1134.

Gracie WA, Ransohoff DF: Medical intelligence: The natural history of silent gallstones; the innocent gallstone is not a myth. *N Engl J Med* 1982; 307:798–800.

Greene MH, Boice JD, Greer BE, Blessing JA, Dembo AJ: Acute nonlymphocytic leukemia after therapy with alkylating agents for ovarian cancer: A study of five randomized clinical trials. *N Engl J Med* 1982; 307:1416–1421.

Greenland S, Thomas DC: On the need for the rare disease assumption in case-control studies. *Am J Epidemiol* 1982; 116:547–553.

Herbst AL, Ulfelder H, Poskanzer DC: Adenocarcinoma of the vagina: Association of maternal stilbestrol therapy with tumor appearance in young women. *N Engl J Med* 1971; 284:878–881.

Hoover R, Fraumeni FJ: Risk of cancer in renal-transplant recipients. *Lancet* 1973; 2:55–57.

Hoover R, Glass A, Finkle WD, Azevedo D, Milne K: Conjugated estrogens and breast cancer risk in women. *JNCI* 1981; 4:815–820.

Horwitz RI, Feinstein AR: Alternative analytic methods for case-control studies of estrogens and endometrial cancer. *N Engl J Med* 1978; 299:1089–1094.

Jick H, Hunter JR, Dinan BJ, Madsen S, Stergachis A: Sedating drugs and automobile accidents leading to hospitalization. *Am J Public Health* 1981; 71:1399–1400.

Jick H, Walter AM, Watkins RN, D'Ewart DC, Hunter JR, Danford A, Madsen S, Dinan BJ, Rothman KJ: Replacement estrogens and breast cancer. *Am J Epidemiol* 1980; 112:586–594.

Kelsey JL, Fischer DB, Holford TR, LiVolsi VA, Mostow ED, Goldenberg IS, White C: Exogenous estrogens and other factors in the epidemiology of breast cancer. *JNCI* 1981; 67:327–333.

Lanier AP, Noller KL, Decker DG, Elveback LR, Kurland LT: Cancer and stilbestrol: A follow-up of 1,719 persons exposed to estrogens in utero and born 1943–1959. *Mayo Clin Proc* 1973; 48:793–799.

MacMahon B, Pugh TF: *Epidemiology: Principles and Methods.* Bsoton, Little, Brown and Company, 1970.

Mann JI, Inman WHW: Oral contraceptives and death from myocardial infarction. *Br Med J* 1975; 2:245–248.

Marks JS, Halpin TJ: Guillain-Barre Syndrome in recipients of A/New Jersey influenza vaccine. *JAMA* 1980; 243:2490–2494.

Meade TW, Greenberg G, Thompson SG: Progestogens and cardiovascular reactions associated with oral contraceptives and a comparison of the safety of 50- and 30-g oestrogen preparations. *Br Med J* 1980; 1157–1161.

Messer J, Reitman D, Sacks HS, Smith H, Chalmers TC: Association of adrenocorticosteroid therapy and peptic-ulcer disease. *N Engl J Med* 1983; 309:21–24.

Miller RR: Drug surveillance utilizing epidemiologic methods: A report from the Boston Collaborative Drug Surveillance Program. *Am J Hosp Pharm* 1973; 30:584–592.

Mitchell AA, Goldman P, Shapiro S, Slone D: Drug utilization and reported adverse reactions in hospitalized children. *Am J Epidemiol* 1979; 110:196–204.

Myers BD, Ross J, Newton L, Luetscher J, Perlroth M: Cyclosporine-associated chronic nephropathy. *N Engl J Med* 1984; 311:699–729.

Reimer RR, Hoover R, Fraumeni JF, Young RC: Acute leukemia after alkylating-agent therapy of ovarian cancer. *N Engl J Med* 1977; 297:177–181.

Rosenberg L, Mitchell AA, Parsells JL, Pashayan H, Louik C, Shapiro S: Lack of relation of oral clefts to diazepam use during pregnancy. *N Engl J Med* 1983; 309:1282–1285.

Ross RK, Paganini-Hill A, Gerkins VR, Mack TM, Pfeffer R, Arthur M, Henderson BE: A case-control study of menopausal estrogen therapy and breast cancer. *JAMA* 1980; 243:1635–1639.

Schlesselman JJ: *Case-control studies* New York, Oxford University Press, 1982.

Shiono PH, Mills JL: Oral clefts and diazepam use during pregnancy. *N Engl J Med* 1984; 311:919–920.

Silverberg SG, Makowski EL, Roche WD: Endometrial carcinoma in women under 40 years of age. *Cancer* 1977; 39:592–598.

Skegg DCG, Doll R: Record linkage for drug monitoring. *J Epidemiol Community Health* 1981; 35:25–31.

Skegg DCG, Richards SM, Doll R: Minor tranquilisers and road accidents. *Br Med J* 1979; 1:917–919.

Slone D, Jick H, Lewis GP, Shapiro S, Miettinen OS: Intravenously given ethacrynic acid and gastrointestinal bleeding: A finding resulting from comprehensive drug surveillance. *JAMA* 1969; 209:1668–1671.

Walker AM, Jick H, Hunter JR, Danford A, Watkins RN, Alhadeff L, Rothman KJ: Vasectomy and non-fatal myocrdial infarction. *Lancet* 1981; 1:13–15.

Weiss NS, Sayvetz TA: Incidence of endometrial cancer in relation to the use of oral contraceptives. *N Engl J Med* 1980; 302:551–554.

7 Natural History of Illness

Studies of the natural history of illness measure health outcomes in persons with a symptom, sign, or condition who are not receiving a therapy that influences the presence or rate of these outcomes. Results obtained from natural history studies are put to use in several important ways.

Natural history studies permit the development of rational strategies for attempting the early detection of untoward consequences in person who have the symptom/sign/condition under study. For example, knowledge of the rate at which various early forms of cervical intraepithelial neoplasia progress either to later forms or to invasive cervical cancer would have an important bearing on determing the frequency with which women having early intraepithelial neoplasia should undergo cytological rescreening of the cervix. Similarly, in patients who have undergone surgery for peptic ulcer disease, the decision to conduct periodic endoscopic surveillance of the gastric remnant so that early cancer can be identified and treated depends heavily on these patients' actual incidence of gastric cancer.

Natural history studies point to the need for treatment of the condition that is present (and the evaluation of the efficacy of that treatment). For example, it is uncertain how aggressive one should be in treating asymptomatic patients who are discovered to have hypercalcemia on routine examination and who upon further testing are found to have elevated levels of parathyroid hormone but no other apparent cause of hypercalcemia. The results of studies that document subsequent morbidity and mortality in such patients can serve as a guide as to whether parathyroidectomy should be considered, or whether it is safe to adopt a conservative approach. Another therapeutic question with no clear answer at present is whether or not to place tympanostomy tubes in the ears of children who have middle ear effusion following acute otitis media. Since children with such effusion show some degree of conductive hearing loss, and since there is reason to believe that conductive hearing loss adversely impairs learning, one might surmise that the presence of effusion over a number of weeks and months could lead to impaired development of speech and language in children. However, before incurring the hazard and expense associated with the placement of tympanostomy tubes, it would be important to know if, and to what extent, persistent effusion actually is associated with retardation in the development of speech and language.

With respect to treatment decisions, there is still another function served by studies of natural history. For practical reasons, randomized controlled trials and other studies of therapeutic efficacy cannot be conducted in all segments of the population. Inevitably, to maximize the internal validity of the study, there are certain entry criteria that potential subjects must meet, whether those criteria are based on demographic, disease, or other characteristics. You would like to know if the measurement of treatment efficacy obtained in these formal studies pertains to those of your patients who do not meet the entry criteria. If, in patients who do and do not match the characteristics of the earlier study subjects, the symptom/sign/condition bears the same relationship to the occurrence of the outcome that you would like to prevent, you should feel comfortable about generalizing the results from one patient group to the other.

Example. Randomized controlled trials conducted in hypertensive white and black men under 70 years of age showed antihypertensive therapy to be efficacious in reducing mortality from cardiovascular disease (Hypertension and Detection Follow-up Program Cooperative Group, 1979). You have two patients with high blood pressure, a 64-year-old Japanese-American man and an 81-year-old Caucasian man. Can you expect antihypertensive therapy to be similarly efficacious in them?

There have been no studies of the efficacy of antihypertensive therapy similar to the one cited that were conducted with Japanese-American or elderly men. So, to begin to answer this question, you turn to studies of natural history, that is, studies relating mortality from cardiovascular disease to blood pressure level in Japanese and elderly men. You find that mortality among Japanese-Americans is strongly related to blood pressure (Yano et al., 1984), but that in the elderly the situation is uncertain (Mitchell, 1983). Based on these data, you might elect not to treat your 81-year-old patient.

Even in the absence of any further detection or therapuetic measures, the results of studies of natural history enable the health care provider to counsel his or her patient by providing a description of possible outcomes that can result from the condition, and of the likelihood with which they will occur.

STUDY DESIGNS FOR MEASURING NATURAL HISTORY

Most commonly, persons with a given symptom/sign/condition are monitored for the occurrence of the outcome(s) of interest, and the rate of incidence is compared with that in a similarly monitored group of unaffected persons and/or the population as a whole. Follow-up (cohort) studies of this type may either be prospective or retrospective, even as follow-up studies that evaluate diagnostic tests or therapy can be. For example, beginning in 1975 the investigators in the Greater Boston Otitis Media Study Group Monitored prospectively the occurrence of acute episodes of middle ear disease and the presence of middle ear effusion in a cohort of newborn infants (Teele et al., 1984). The development of speech and language in a sample of these children was then evaluated 3 years later. By way of contrast, investigators at the Kaiser Foundation Health Plan studied the natural history of hypercalcemia using a retrospective approach. In 1976, they identified members who had had at least two abnormal calcium values obtained during a multiphasic health examination during the years 1964 to 1973 (Rubinoff et al., 1983). These patients' medical records were reviewed to eliminate subjects with a "secondary" cause of hypercalcemia and to determine the occurrence of a wide variety of symptoms and illnesses through 1976.

To determine if the rate of an outcome in patients with a particular symptom/sign/condition is atypical, a comparison with the rate in other persons is necessary. The comparison group is often found in the source population from which those with the symptom/sign/condition were identified. For example, the development of speech and language at the age of 3 years in the children who often had middle ear effusion was compared with that in children from the same study population who had experienced little or no effusion. The patients with hypercalcemia were compared, for subsequent symptoms and illnesses, with another group of persons who had normal serum calcium levels during the multiphasic examination.

Alternatively, in some natural history follow-up studies it is necessary to obtain comparison data from outside the study cohort itself. For example, the rate of subsequent gastric cancer among residents of Olmsted County, Minnesota, who underwent surgery for peptic ulcer at the Mayo Clinic was compared with that of all Olmsted County residents (Schafer et al., 1983).

It is also possible to undertake case-control studies that evaluate natural history. These case-control studies begin by identifying patients who have sustained the outcome or endpoint of interest. The patients are compared, for the presence of earlier symptoms signs/conditions, with otherwise similar persons who did not sustain this outcome. For example, several investigators were interested in determining the extent to which various nonspecific respiratory and gastrointestinal symptoms predict the occurrence of sudden and unexpected death among infants. They identified infants who had died suddenly, and, for comparison, selected healthy infants from birth records in the community in which the cases had resided (Stanton et al., 1978). Parents of both cases and controls were interviewed about the presence of symptoms in the several days prior to death (or at a corresponding point for controls).

Case-control studies of natural history do not provide directly the rates of a particular outcome in relation to the presence of a symptom/sign/condition, for in case-control studies one determines only the frequency of these antecedents in persons who have developed the outcome. Nonetheless, as was seen in Chapter 6, with some additional information on the incidence of the outcome, the data from case-control studies can be used to help estimate these rates.

ISSUES IN THE ANALYSIS AND INTERPRETATION OF NATURAL HISTORY STUDIES

An Association Between a Condition and a Particular Outcome May Not be Indicative of a Cause–Effect Relationship

In the context of natural history studies, the word "cause" means that, if the patient's condition were to be eliminated, his or her chances of developing the untoward outcome would be reduced. It is necessary to reach a verdict of "causal" or "noncausal" for many suspected antecedents of untoward outcomes because usually there will be less interest in detecting or treating the symptom/sign/condition if it will have no effect on the occurrence of the outcome.

Before concluding that a given condition predisposes a patient to an altered risk of a given outcome, one must at the very least be convinced that the condition *preceded* the outcome, and not the other way around. For example, in a number of studies, persons with low levels of serum cholesterol have been noted to experience an increased rate of cancer. Detracting from the hypothesis of a causal relationship between low levels of serum cholesterol and cancer is the suspicion that occult cancer can cause a fall in the serum cholesterol concentration. This theory arises from the observation in several (though not all) of these studies that the low cholesterol–cancer association is present for several years following the cholesterol measurement, but not thereafter (Salmond et al., 1985).

> *Example.* When conducting their follow-up study of the possible relationship between primary hypogammaglobulinemia and the subsequent occurrence of cancer, Kinlen et al. (1985) wanted to exclude the possibility that such an association could be attributable to immunosuppressive activity of an occult malignancy. Thus, they restricted their analysis to cancers that occurred after the first 2 years following diagnosis of hypogammaglobulinemia. Even though this reduced the number of study subjects—61 of the original 377 patients did not survive 2 years—their finding of a fivefold increased cancer risk offers an interpretation that is considerably clearer than had they started to tabulate cancer incidence immediately upon each subject's entry into the study.

Other criteria used for inferring causal relationships were elaborated in Chapter 6. Of particular relevance to studies of natural history are the criteria concerning the strength of the association and the biologic plausibility of a causal connection between the condition and the outcome. To illustrate the ways in which these criteria are put to use, let's consider the interpretation of the reports of two different studies of natural history.

In the first study, patients with untreated aortic insufficiency were followed and found to have many-fold increased rate of the development of angina, congestive heart failure, and mortality (Spagnuolo et al., 1971). In the second study, patients with a carotid bruit were found to have a twofold increased rate of stroke (Wolf et al., 1981). The question: In patients with aortic insufficiency or with a carotid bruit, to what extent would surgical intervention improve this natural history? To answer: In each instance we must judge first whether the valvular or arterial lesion played a causal role in the development of the untoward outcomes, or whether there was some underlying condition that gave rise both to the lesion and to the subsequent events. While all the patients with aortic insufficiency in that study of Spagnuolo et al. had previously had an attack of rheumatic fever, there has been enough experience with the sequelae of rheumatic fever in the absence of aortic insufficiency to rule out the possibility that the rheumatic fever per se played an important role in the development of angina, heart failure, and so on. On the other hand, the underlying condition that most commonly gives rise to carotid bruits in older persons, arteriosclerotic vascular disease, is associated with an increased risk of stroke even in the absence of a carotid bruit. Indeed, when Wolf et al. analyzed their data according to the vascular territory in which each stroke occurred, they found it bore little relation to the vessel in which the bruit had been present. This last analysis provided convincing evidence that the underlying condition, rather than the lesion that produced the physical sign, was playing a causal role in the development of stroke, which argues against performing surgery designed only to remedy the source of the bruit.

The Relation of the Symptom/Sign/Condition to the Occurrence of the Outcome May Not be the Same for all Categories of Patients

Most symptoms/signs/conditions have a natural history that varies considerably from patient to patient. Some persons with hypertension rapidly develop ocular and renal damage: others seem to suffer no ill effects. Among women with metastatic breast cancer, some are destined to die soon, while in others the condition may persist for more than a decade.

One of the goals of natural history studies is the ability to indicate, among patients with a certain symptom/sign/condition, which ones will do well and which ones will not. To set out to accomplish the goal, it is necessary only to monitor the separate natural histories of subgroups of patients defined according to characteristics of the symptom/sign/condition or of the patients themselves.

Example. Patients with unruptured intracranial aneurysms were followed to ascertain the natural history of these lesions (Wiebers et al., 1981). Eight of 29 aneurysms 1 cm or greater in diameter ruptured during the follow-up period (averaging 8 years per patient), in contrast to 0 of 44 lesions rupturing that were less than 1 cm in diameter. The authors concluded that prompt intracranial surgery should be restricted to patients with aneurysms 1 cm or larger in diameter.

Example. Patients with extensive ulcerative colitis (*n* = 303) were monitored for the occurrence of colorectal cancer (Lennard-Jones et al., 1983). In the 914 patient-years that accrued within the first 10 years of the onset of symptoms, no carcinomas developed. In contrast, 13 carcinomas were diagnosed in the 1,167 patient-years that accrued beyond the first 10 years of the illness. The authors recommended that, once the duration of symptoms reaches 10 years, patients with ulcerative colitis should undergo either careful follow-up evaluation or proctocolectomy.

Example. Teele et al. (1984) monitored a cohort of children from birth for the occurrence of otitis media and middle ear effusion, and then measured the children's development of speech and language at age 3 years. The duration of middle ear effusion during the first year of life, but not during the next 2 years, was associated with low performance on the speech and language tests. If confirmed, these results should have a bearing on the age at which it is deemed appropriate to treat middle ear effusion in children with tympanostomy tubes.

Example. Men with angina pectoris were found to have a mortality rate three to four times that of men without any manifestation of coronary heart disease (Frank et al., 1973). The size of the excess rate was similar in men of different ages but was increased considerably in hypertensive men and those in whom an electrocardiogram showed evidence of coronary heart disease. Indeed, among men with angina whose blood pressure was normal and who had a normal electrocardiogram, the mortality rate was only slightly above that of men without angina. Mortality differences based on these characteristics and on even more impressive ones based on findings at coronary arteriography can play an important role in a physician's recommendation as to whether or not coronary artery surgery should be performed.

Case-control studies are more often used to delineate subgroups of patients with a given symptom/sign/condition who are at altered risk of the outcome than they are used to study other aspects of natural history. For example, Dornon et al. (1982) sought to characterize insulin-dependent diabetics who are resistant to the development of retinopathy. They compared 40 persons with long-standing diabetes (average duration 30 years) who had normal eyes with diabetic controls who had retinopathy, matched for duration and age at onset of diabetes, with regard to such characteristics as weight, blood pressure, and smoking habits. (Indirectly, they also attempted to measure the efficacy of hypoglycemic therapy by contrasting the blood glucose levels between the groups during the years following the diagnosis of diabetes.) In a similar way, a case-control study was conducted to determine the factors that predict a "benign" course in multiple sclerosis (Clark et al., 1982).

The Nature of the Study Subjects May Restrict the Generalization of Observations

When considering to what extent associations found in studies of natural history can be generalized to other patient groups, criteria similar to those espoused earlier for studies of therapy (Chapter 4 and 6) are employed. But to generalize regarding the rate at which subsequent outcomes occur, it is also necessary to take into account the similarity of study and reference populations with regard to the point in the natural history of the condition at which members of the two populations are identified. When counselling patients about their prognosis, for instance, you would want to base your appraisal on data from patients "like" them, especially in terms of where they are in the course of the condition. For example, the expected consequences of your patient's hypercalcemia, detected fortuitously from a battery of blood chemistry tests, may differ considerably from those of patients whose hypercalcemia was detected after symptoms (e.g., renal colic) led them to seek medical care.

> *Example.* The study of mortality rates in men with angina pectoris (Frank et al., 1973) was conducted in a large prepaid health care plan. Medical records were reviewed during a 4-year period to identify men aged 25 to 64 years with symptoms or signs suggestive of angina; these men were asked to attend a special examination. At that time a detailed history was taken, and from this history a judgment was made as to whether the subject did or did not have angina. Mortality rates in the men with angina were calculated, but these rates would not necessarily apply to men with newly diagnosed angina. The study subjects, being a sample of cases prevalent during a 4-year period, no doubt included a number of cases well along in their natural history, the longevity of which might be expected to be less than that of new cases. (Mortality rates calculated in this study are less likely to be misleading when used for another purpose—the comparison of subgroups of men with angina to identify those at particularly high or low risk of death.)

QUESTIONS, CHAPTER 7

7-1. A group of investigators (Gresham et al., 1975) sought to determine "the magnitude and pattern of long-term stroke disability, [to provide] the basis for planning continuing care programs for surviving stroke victims and [to permit] a more accurate prognosis to be made for the individual patient in terms of eventual functional recovery." From the Framingham cohort, a group of more than 5,000 persons monitored for the occurrence of cardiovascular disease since the early 1950s, they identified during 1972 to 1974 the 123 survivors of the 313 persons who had sustained a stroke in the prior 20 or so years. They evaluated each subject in terms of his or her functional disability and need for institutional care, and compared them in these respects with other living members of the cohort, matched for age and sex. The results were as follows: 31% of the stroke survivors versus 8% of the controls were dependent on others for the activities of daily living; 14% of the stroke survivors versus 2% of the controls were residing in a nursing home or chronic-disease hospital. Did the study accomplish the stated aims of the investigators?

7-2.   To test the hypothesis that the presence of endometriosis predisposes women to infertility, a group of investigators conducted a case-control study (Strathy et al., 1982). They reviewed the medical records of 100 women who underwent diagnostic laparoscopy for infertility and, applying the standards of The American Fertility Society, classified 21 as having endometriosis.

The investigators were able to show that a clinical diagnosis of endometriosis was neither a sensitive nor a specific means of determining endometriosis as diagnosed by laparoscopy. Thus, the choice of a control group posed a problem, for it was necessary to identify fertile women who also had undergone laparoscopy. They decided to select 200 women, similar in age to the cases but otherwise selected at random, from among those who underwent laparoscopy for tubal ligation during the same period. Based on the findings reported in the records of these control subjects, only four were deemed to have endometriosis.

    a. From these data, can you estimate the risk of infertility in women with endometriosis relative to that in other women? If so, what is that relative risk? if not, why not?

    b. Critics of the study claimed that, despite their efforts, the investigators were unable to achieve comparable ascertainment of endometriosis in cases and controls. What do you think was the basis for this criticism?

ANSWERS

7-1.   The study as designed was capable of providing an answer only to the question, "Do persons who have survived a stroke have a greater degree of disability than other persons?" (It is arguable whether a formal study was needed to provide the obvious answer.) The design left unevaluated the issue of the natural history of stroke that the authors had intended to address. To have done so would have required monitoring survival and functional status in all 313 persons from the time their stroke occurred. This task would have been more difficult than evaluating survivors in 1972 to 1974, and no doubt information regarding functional status of victims in the 1950s and 1960s would have been imprecise and in some cases unavailable. But such a design at least would have been responsive to the question the authors had posed.

7-2.

		Infertile women	Controls
Endometriosis:	Yes	21	4
	No	79	196

The relative risk can be estimated as $21 \div 79/4 \div 196 = 13.0$.

b. The critics might have argued that, with regard to finding endometriosis, laparoscopy done as part of an investigation of a woman's infertility might not be comparable to laparoscopy done to perform a tubal ligation. This especially could be true if (as in this study) no attempt was made to standardize the ascertainment method in cases and controls, which could lead to a substantial overestimation of the risk of infertility associated with endometriosis.

REFERENCES

Clark VA, Detels R, Visscher BR, Valdiviezo NL, Malmgren RM, Dudley JP. Factors associated with a malignant or benign course of multiple sclerosis. *JAMA* 1982; 248:856–860.

Dornan T, Mann JI, Turner R: Factors protective against retinopathy in insulin-dependent diametics free of retinopathy for 30 years. *Br Med J* 1982; 285:1073–1077.

Frank CW, Weinblatt E, Shapiro S: Angina pectoris in men: Prognostic significance of selected medical factors. *Circulation* 1973; 47:509–517.

Gresham GE, Fitzpatrick TE, Wolf PA, McNamara PM, Kannel WB, Dawber TR: Residual disability in survivors of stroke—The Framingham Study *Engl J Med* 1975; 293:954–956.

Hypertension and Detection Follow-up Program Cooperative Group: Five-year findings of the hypertension detection and follow-up program: II. Mortality by race, sex and age. *JAMA* 1979; 242:2572–2577.

Kinlen LJ, Webster ADB, Bird AG, Haile R, Peto J, Soothill JF, Thompson RA: Prospective study of cancer in patients with hypogammaglobulinaemia. *Lancet* 1985; 1:263–266.

Lennard-Jones JE, Morson BC, Ritchie JK, Williams CB: Cancer surveillance in ulcerative colitis: Experience over 15 years. *Lancet* 1983; 2:149–152.

Mitchell JRA: Blood pressure and mortality in the very old. *Lancet* 1983; 2:1248.

Rubinoff H, McCarthy N, Hiatt RA: Hypercalcemia: Long-term follow-up with matched controls. *J Chron Dis* 1983; 36:859–868.

Salmond CE, Beaglehole R, Prior IAM: Are low cholesterol values associated with excess mortality? *Br Med J* 1985; 290:422–424.

Schafer LW, Larson DE, Melton J. Higgins JA, Ilstrup DM: The risk of gastric carcinoma after surgical treatment for benign ulcer disease. *N Engl J Med* 1983; 309:1210–1212.

Spagnuolo M, Kloth H, Taranta A, Doyle E, Pasternack B: Natural history of rheumatic aortic regurgitation. *Circulation* 1971; 44:368–379.

Stanton AN, Downham MAPS, Oakley JR, Emery JL, Knowelden J: Terminal symptoms in children dying suddenly and unexpectedly at home. *Br Med J* 1978; 2:1249–1251.

Strathy JH, Molgaard CA, Coulam CB, et al: Endometriosis and infertility: A laparoscopic study of endometriosis among fertile and infertile women. *Fertil Steril* 1982; 38:667–672.

Teele DW, Klein JO, Rosner BA, The Greater Boston Otitis Media Study Group: Otitis media with effusion during the first three years of life and development of speech and language. *Pediatrics* 1984; 74:282–287.

Wiebers DO, Whisnant JP, O'Fallon WM: The natural history of unruptured intra-
    cranial aneurysms. *N Engl J Med* 1981; 304:696–698.
Wolf PA, Kannel WB, Sorlie P, McNamara P: Asymptomatic carotid bruit and risk
    of stroke: The Framingham Study. *JAMA* 1981; 245:1442–1445.
Yano K, Reed DM, McGee DL: Ten-year incidence of coronary heart disease in the
    Honolulu heart program: Relationship to biologic and lifestyle characteris-
    tics. *Am J Epidemiol* 1984; 119:653–666.

APPENDIX **Some Methodologic Tools Useful in the Planning and Analysis of Clinical Epidemiologic Research**

ESTIMATION OF THE NUMBER OF SUBJECTS NEEDED IN A STUDY

Let's say you are interested in determining if a particular new form of therapy improves survival following myocardial infarction. You have gone to the trouble of organizing and carrying out a study that compares mortality in persons who did and did not receive the therapy. In analyzing the results, you find a lower mortality in the treated group, but a test for statistical significance indicates that the difference between the rate in that group and the rate in control patients easily could have occurred by chance. Thus, you are left with two possible interpretations: (a) The new treatment truly had no effect, and it *was* just by chance that a difference emerged. (b) There really was a benefit from the treatment, but it was not large enough to be detected as "significant" in a study this size.

The finding of a positive but not statistically significant result occurs thousands of times each year in the medical literature. (Pity those who must interpret such a finding, as if there were not already enough uncertainties for them in the management of their patients!) Sometimes this ambiguous situation cannot be avoided, but the best way to try to avoid it is by planning a large enough study at the outset.

To start, it is necessary to make some guesses as to what the study results might look like. The single most important piece of information needed is the size of the expected difference between the groups being compared. The larger the difference, the smaller will be the number of subjects required. For example, if a new treat-

129

ment for myocardial infarction were to result in a survival of 95% in a subgroup in whom the survival would otherwise be 5%, not too many subjects would have to be enrolled before the benefit would be deemed statistically significant. Also needed is an estimate of the frequency with which an unfavorable outcome will occur in the control group, and a decision regarding the chances you are willing to take for the study to result in a conclusion that is incorrect.

At first glance, it might seem that much of the above information could never be known in advance. Fortunately, it is not necessary to "know" any of it, but merely to make some reasonable guesses. After all, it is only for planning purposes that the number of study subjects is being estimated. Differences of 10 to 20% in the estimated number of subjects that result from the use of incorrect assumptions are almost never of any real importance.

Specifically, in any study in which two groups are being compared (e.g., treated vs. untreated), it would be necessary to enroll the following number of patients (n) in the treated[1] group:

$$n = \frac{(Z_\alpha + Z_\beta)^2 \times \dfrac{R+1}{R} \times p(1-p)}{(p_1 - p_2)^2}$$

where Z_α quantifies the probability of finding a relationship between treatment and the occurrence of a favorable outcome when none is truly present ("α error") and Z_β quantifies the probability of failing to find such a relationship when an effect of a specified size actually is present ("β error"). Values of Z_α and Z_β that correspond to selected probabilities are as follows:

Probability of error	Z_α (two-tailed test)	Z_β
0.05	1.96	1.645
0.10	1.645	1.28
0.20	1.28	0.84
0.50	0.675	0.00

The particular pair of values chosen depends on the thoroughness with which the investigator would like to exclude the possibility that

---

[1]In a case-control study, in which it is the presence or absence of therapy that is being ascertained, n is the number of "cases" (for example, the number of deaths following myocardial infarction).

an unfortunate choice of sample (from the universe of all possible samples of subjects that could be drawn to address this question) has led to the "wrong" result. The more thorough the exclusion, the larger will be the values chosen for Z_α and Z_β, and the larger will be the number of subjects required. Commonly chosen values for Z_α and Z_β are 1.96 and 1.28, respectively, or 1.96 and 0.84.

R in the equation is the ratio of nontreated subjects to treated subjects. Often this ratio is close to one for, given a fixed *total* number of subjects, a ratio of one will provide the most statistical power. If the total is not fixed, however (e.g., in a nonexperimental study), it is possible to achieve some reduction in the number of treated subjects needed by increasing the number of nontreated subjects.

p_1 and p_2 in the equation are the respective cumulative probabilities of an unfavorable outcome in the untreated and treated groups:

$$p = \frac{p_2 + Rp_1}{1 + R}$$

Example. Given medical care currently available, you expect 30% of a poor-risk subgroup of patients who have sustained a myocardial infarction to die within 1 year. You believe a new therapeutic intervention would reduce this to 20%, and maybe even to 15%. You are planning a randomized controlled trial to evaluate the intervention. How large should it be?

Calculate n for each level of mortality reduction to get a range of values. First, for $p_2 = 0.20$:

$Z_\alpha = 1.96$, $Z_\beta = 1.28$
$R = 1$ (one patient without the treatment for every one that receives it)
$p_1 = 0.30$

$$p = \frac{0.20 + 1(0.30)}{1 + 1} = 0.25,\ 1 - p = 0.75$$

$$n = \frac{(1.96 + 1.28)^2 \times \dfrac{1 + 1}{1} \times 0.25(0.75)}{(0.3 - 0.2)^2} = 394$$

Next, for $p_2 = 0.15$:

$$p = \frac{0.15 + (0.30)}{1 + 1} = 0.225$$

$$n = \frac{(1.96 + 1.28)^2 \times \dfrac{1 + 1}{1} \times 0.225(0.775)}{(0.3 - 0.15)^2} = 163$$

Thus, if the 1-year mortality reduction associated with this new therapy is 0.30 − 0.15 = 0.15, 163 treated and 163 untreated patients will be needed to determine the difference reliably. If the mortality reduction is smaller, only 0.30 − 0.20 = 0.10, a far larger number of patients per group, 394, will be required.

The above example illustrates the fact that small changes in the size of the difference being investigated have a striking impact on the size of the study needed to detect that difference. When designing a study, it is always a good idea to perform these calculations over a range of plausible differences in the occurrence of endpoints between the treated and untreated groups. It may be that, over the whole of the plausible range, the number of subjects needed is beyond your means to assemble.

What if the number of subjects is fixed before the investigation begins? Perhaps the study involves a chart review of all patients with myocardial infarction who, during a defined period of time in certain institutions, did and did not receive a certain intervention. In this situation, it is possible to rearrange the equation to estimate the ability ("power") of the investigation to evaluate a specific hypothesis concerning the degree of efficacy of the intervention.

Let's say there are about 900 patients for whom charts are available for review, and it is estimated that about one-third of these patients received the therapy under study. The first step is to stipulate a range of plausible outcomes of the study, for example, a range of differences in mortality between the groups that did and did not receive the therapy. If, as before, the expected 1-year mortality in the untreated patients is 30%, perhaps it is felt that if the therapy had been effective the corresponding mortality in the treated patients could have been as low as 15% or as high as 25%. One can then calculate the probability of committing a β error, that is, the probability of failing to find a difference of each of these magnitudes if one were present:

$$Z_\beta = \frac{\sqrt{n} \times (p_1 - p_2)}{\sqrt{\dfrac{R+1}{R} \times p(1-p)}} - Z_\alpha$$

For $p_2 = 0.25$:

$Z_\alpha = 1.96$

$R = 2$ (600 untreated ÷ 300 treated)

$p_1 = 0.30$

$$p = \frac{0.25 + 2(0.30)}{1 + 2} = 0.283, 1 - p = 0.717$$

$$Z_\beta = \frac{\sqrt{300} \times (0.30 - 0.25)}{\sqrt{\dfrac{2 + 1}{2} \times 0.283\,(0.717)}} - 1.96 = -0.39$$

For $p_2 = 0.15$:

$$p = \frac{0.15 + 2(0.30)}{1 + 2} = 0.25, 1 - p = 0.75$$

$$Z_\beta = \frac{\sqrt{300} \times (0.30 - 0.15)}{\sqrt{\dfrac{2 + 1}{2} \times 0.25(0.75)}} - 1.96 = 2.939$$

To find the probability of failing to detect the respective mortality differences between treated and untreated patients, simply refer to the table on p. 130 (or for a more precise figure, the table of areas of the normal curve in a statistics text). There would be a high probability ($> 50\%$) that a study of 900 patients would be unable to discern a mortality difference of $0.30 - 0.25 = 0.05$. On the other hand, if the difference were really as great as $0.30 - 0.15 = 0.15$, then the chances of failing to find it as statistically significant would be far less than 5%.

The statistical power of a study to detect a difference of a designated size is defined as $(1 - \beta) \times 100$. Thus, while the above study had a great deal of power ($> 95\%$) to evaluate the hypothesis that the mortality reduction was $0.30 - 0.15 = 0.15$, its power was less than 50% to assess the hypothesis that the difference was $0.30 - 0.25 = 0.05$.

Often the study outcome to be measured is not a dichotomous one (e.g., recovered vs. not recovered) but rather a characteristic for which there are many levels (e.g., blood pressure, weight, arterial Po_2). In such situations, it is also possible to estimate the number of subjects required to reliably identify a given change between treatment groups or, for a sample of fixed size, the power of the study to detect that change. The formula used can be found in most textbooks of biostatistics (for example, Colton, 1974); it is analogous to the one presented above, but requires explicit estimation of the standard deviation of the characteristic in the population under study.

CONTROLLING FOR THE INFLUENCE OF CONFOUNDING VARIABLES

In clinical epidemiology, a confounding variable is one whose influence distorts the true relationship between an intervention (or a patient characteristic) and the outcome of disease. For instance, in a nonexperimental study of the ability of local excision ("lumpectomy") and radical mastectomy to prevent death from breast cancer, the comparison would probably be distorted by the fact that women with large tumors (who thus have a relatively poor prognosis) would be present disproportionately among those in whom a radical mastectomy were performed. The confounding variable would be tumor size.

A variable's confounding influence can be controlled in one of three ways:

1. By restricting selection of subjects for study to a single "level" of the confounder. Thus, in the evaluation of surgery for breast cancer, it might be possible to confine the study to a narrow range of small tumor sizes within which there is little or no variation in mortality rates.
2. By choosing subjects in such a way as to make the groups being compared identical with respect to the presence of the confounding variable. Thus, to every woman who underwent local excision of her breast tumor, one could match a woman with a tumor of the same size but who underwent radical mastectomy.
3. By artificially forcing ("adjusting"), in the analysis, the groups being compared to have the same status concerning the confounding variable. The results are presented (see below) to answer a question such as this: If the distribution of tumor size in the group that underwent local excision had really been the same as that in the group that underwent radical mastectomy, what would have been the difference in breast cancer mortality?

Each of the three methods is valid. The choice in a particular study is usually made on the basis of practicality, after considering the answers to questions like the following: After restriction, are there enough subjects to study? How much effort and cost would be involved in matching? If nothing is done until the analysis, will there be enough overlap between groups with respect to the confounding factor so that adjustment will be possible?

Adjustment for Confounding Effects

The remainder of the discussion will focus on the last method (adjustment), partly because of the frequency with which it is called for and partly because it is not as readily understood as are the first two methods.

Example. Let's say that 5 years ago, a drug with a potent β-adrenergic blocking action was introduced. It has now been prescribed by a number of physicians in your community to survivors of acute myocardial infarction (MI), and you would like to know if it has been effective in reducing subsequent cardiac-related mortality in these patients. Through hospital discharge diagnoses, you identify 200 persons who sustained an MI and survived for 72 hours. With the help of the patients' physicians and the state vital statistics office, you determine which of them had received the β-blocker and which of them died during the subsequent 18 months. The results, presented according to whether or not there was evidence of congestive heart failure during the first 72 hours after the MI occurred, are shown in Table A-1.

Overall, there is a 6.1% difference in mortality that favors the group that received the β-blocker. However, you are concerned that there is barely any benefit associated with the drug when the difference is calculated for each of the two subgroups based on heart failure status (none and mild; patients with more severe heart failure would not be given this drug). What accounts for this discrepancy?

The answer is that the overall difference of 6.1% is due to the influence of two factors (for the purposes of this example, we will ignore the possibility—a likely one—that chance has contributed to the difference as well): (a) the true benefit derived from the action of the β-blocker (somewhere between 1.6 and 2.1%) and (b) the distoring (confounding) influence of the variable congestive heart failure in this analysis. The distortion occurs because patients with mild congestive heart failure, itself a risk factor for cardiac mortality, are less likely to be prescribed the drug than are patients with no heart

Table A-1. Mortality in the 18 Months Following Myocardial Infarction, by Treatment and Congestive Heart Failure Status

Congestive heart failure	β-blocker prescribed[a]			β-blocker not prescribed			Difference (% mortality)
	MI patients	Cardiac deaths	% deaths	MI patients	Cardiac deaths	% deaths	
Mild	18	4	22.2	42	10	23.8	1.6
None	99	10	10.1	41	5	12.2	2.1
Mild + None	117	14	12.0	83	15	18.1	6.1

[a]During the first 72 hours. For simplicity, it is assumed that β-blocker therapy would not be initiated after this time.

failure: the cardiac mortality in patients not receiving the β-blocker was 10 in 42, or 23.8%, in those with mild heart failure, and 5 in 41, or 12.2%, in those without heart failure. The occurrence of mild congestive heart failure following MI in patients prescribed the β-blocker was 18 in 117, or 15.4%, and in patients not prescribed the β-blocker, 42 in 83, or 50.6%. Thus, the cardiac mortality in the group receiving the β-blocker was spuriously low because the group contained a high proportion of patients at relatively low risk, those without heart failure.

To discern the "true" benefit associated with β-blocker use, it is only necessary to examine the results separately for patients with and without heart failure. The distortion due to the existence of unequal proportions of patients with heart failure in the treated and untreated groups cannot occur unless the data are lumped together without considering this risk factor for cardiac mortality. However, as the number of categories of the confounding variable and/or the number of confounding variables grow, the failure to present some sort of summary result will make it increasingly hard to understand and communicate the findings of the study.

The means by which a summary but unconfounded result can be obtained is called *adjustment*. Adjustment "forces" the treatment groups being compared to have the same pattern of other risk factors (e.g., heart failure), no matter how different they may actually be. The mortality in each subgroup (e.g., mild heart failure, no heart failure) is "weighted" identically among treated and untreated patients.

In the β-blocker example, the adjusted percent mortality in treated and untreated groups, with the distribution of heart failure status chosen arbitrarily to be that of the untreated group, is calculated as follows:

    a. Calculate "weights":
            Proportion with mild heart failure = 42/83 = 0.506
            Proportion with no heart failure   = 41/83 = 0.494
                                                  1.000
    b. Calculate heart failure–specific percent mortality:

Heart failure	β-Blocker–treated	Untreated
Mild	22.2%	23.8%
None	10.1%	12.2%

c. Calculate summary percent mortality weighted identically in both groups:

Heart failure	β-Blocker–treated			Untreated		
	% mortality	Weight	Weighted % mortality	% mortality	Weight	Weighted % mortality
Mild	22.2	0.506	11.23	23.8	0.506	12.04
None	10.1	0.494	4.99	12.2	0.494	6.03
Total (adjusted)			16.2			18.1
Difference (% mortality)				1.9%		

The adjusted difference is 1.9%, quite a "good" summary of the differences of 1.6 and 2.1% (calculated previously) that were found for persons with mild and no heart failure, respectively.

To what extent is the size of the adjusted difference dependent on the particular set of weights used? The same calculation can be performed using weights that arise from the distribution of mild and no heart failure in the β-blocker group, for the combined groups, or for any other distribution. The only restriction is that the sum of the weights equal 1.000:

Basis	Weights		Sum of weights	Adjusted % mortality		Difference (% mortality, adjusted)
	Mild	None		β-Blocker–treated	Untreated	
β-blocker–treated	18/117 = 0.154	99/117 = 0.846	1.000	11.96	13.99	2.0%
Combined	60/200 = 0.300	140/200 = 0.700	1.000	13.73	15.68	1.95%

In this instance the choice of weights makes only a small difference in the adjusted percent mortality, the values of which range from 1.9 to 2.0%.

When Not to Adjust

If the size of the adjusted difference varied to a greater degree with one particular set of weights, it would be inadvisable to adjust: The results of the study should not depend on an arbitrary choice of the investigator! In this instance, it would be necessary to take the time and effort to present the percent mortality difference separately for persons both with and without heart failure.

In practice, it is not necessary to use a variety of weights to determine how much the adjusted result will vary from one set to the next. All that is needed before deciding to adjust is the examination of the percent mortality difference (or whatever measure of outcome is being used in the study) in each of the various groups (e.g., mild vs. no heart failure). If the differences do not vary to a degree that you believe to be important, then adjustment is appropriate and, whatever your selection of weights, the results will be similar.

What is an important degree of variation in the differences, one to which you should pay attention? To a large extent this represents a subjective judgment. In this judgment you will consider the likelihood with which the variation could have occurred by chance, and to what extent the variation "makes sense" in terms of the relevant biology. [Do not expect your colleagues (or reviewers) always to arrive at the same judgment that you did.]

Events that occur *after* the therapy has been given (or, for studies of natural history, after the condition has first been diagnosed) are treated as confounding factors only under unusual circumstances. If you were comparing the mortality of post-MI patients treated with a β-blocker with the mortality of those treated in other ways, you would not control for the presence of congestive heart failure that developed after treatment was initiated (or at a corresponding point for controls). You would be concerned that the development of heart failure in some way may have been due to an effect of the therapy or to its absence, and that forcing the compared groups to be similar with respect to posttreatment heart failure would serve only to reduce the true between-group difference.

Example. A colleague in the Department of Obstetrics and Gynecology is interested in factors that influence the survival of her patients with endometrial cancer. She has data on several hundred such patients, including those relating to estrogen use (both prior to and following diagnosis), stage of disease at diagnosis (e.g., confined to the endometrium, spread to other parts of the uterus, spread beyond the uterus), and survival. Under what circumstances, if any, would you advise her to adjust for "stage of disease at diagnosis" when examining: (a) the relationship between estrogen use *prior to* diagnosis and survival? (b) the relationship between estrogen use *following* diagnosis and survival? You would advise her as follows: (a) Do not adjust for stage of disease, since it is something that has been determined *after* estrogen use. It is possible, for example, that estrogen use could influence survival of endometrial cancer by influencing the stage at which the cancer is detected. By adjusting for stage, you would be negating this effect. (b) Do adjust for stage of disease if users and nonusers of estrogens *following* diagnosis differ with respect to stage. They might well differ— only women with no evidence of tumor following hysterectomy and bilateral oophorectomy could reasonably be considered for estrogen therapy—and so, the failure to adjust could result in a spurious beneficial effect associated with estrogen use.

Rarely, there will be a hypothesis that, to be addressed properly, does require post-therapy events to be adjusted for. We are interested, for example, in determining whether a woman's use of oral contraceptives prior to her first pregnancy predisposes her to an increased risk of breast cancer. We know that because it delays the first pregnancy, the use of the pill (and any other effective contraceptive) leads to a higher incidence of breast cancer. But to learn whether pill use affects risk above and beyond its pregnancy-delaying effects, we must control for "age at first pregnancy." In a case-control study, controls might be matched to cases on the basis of age at first pregnancy. Alternatively, in the absence of matching, this variable could be adjusted for in the analysis.

Alternate Presentation of an Adjusted Result

Sometimes, for descriptive purposes, it is desirable to summarize the results of a study by comparing the number of "observed" events (e.g., deaths, recurrences, complications) in a group of interest with the number that would have been "expected" on the basis of the experience of a control group. This is a particularly clear form of presentation when the observed number is small. So, in the β-blocker study, the observed number of deaths was 14. How can an expected number be calculated to take into account the confounding influence of the congestive heart failure variable?

All that needs to be done is to apply the percent mortality in each subgroup of the untreated patients to the number of treated patients in the subgroups:

Heart failures	Untreated patients (% mortality)	No. of treated patients	Expected no.
Mild	23.8%	18	4.28
None	12.2%	99	12.08
Total			16.4

Since 14 deaths were observed to occur and 16.4 were expected, a small benefit related to the use of the β-blocker is present. Note that the expected number with heart failure status *not* taken into account is 21.2. The difference between the latter and 14 greatly overestimates the efficacy of the drug.

Adjustment of Ratios of Rates or Proportions?

While for many purposes it is the difference between two rates or proportions that you will wish to measure, on occasion the ratio between these will be of importance. When the adjusted rates or proportions have already been calculated to find the difference between them, it is easy to put these same numbers into a fraction. For example, using the percentages from p. 137, the adjusted mortality *ratio* between patients treated without and with a β-blocker would be 18.1%/16.2% = 1.12.

But what if you would like to measure the adjusted relative incidence from a case-control study? Let's say you have determined the frequency of oral contraceptive use in women under age 45 years who died of a myocardial infarction, as well as in controls. In this situation, there are no adjusted rates or proportions to be calculated. All you can do is to estimate the relative incidence, but you would like to do so having adjusted for any characteristics that differ between cases and controls. In the following data, from Mann and Inman (1975), the design of the study produced a greater number of controls than cases only in the younger age group. Since "current" oral contraceptive use was strongly related to a woman's age, failure to adjust for age could lead to a biased estimate of any excess risk.

A commonly used means of calculating the adjusted relative incidence from data from case-control studies is shown in Table A-2 (Mantel and Haenszel, 1959). In this example, note that the relative incidence unadjusted for age would have been $(29 \times 109) \div (19 \times 70) = 2.38$. This value is spuriously low, and results from the presence of a higher proportion of younger women among controls than among cases, younger women being a group in whom current oral contraceptive use is relatively more common.

Alternatives to Adjustment?

Whether you are adjusting for the confounding effects of one or several factors at a time, the process is usually the same. For example, in the study on the efficacy of the new β-blocker, let's say that you want to control for the patient's sex, in addition to controlling

Table A-2. Calculation of Adjusted Relative Incidence from Case-Control Study Data

General Example

Subgroup i

Unintended effect:
Present   Absent

		Present	Absent
Therapy administered:	Yes	a_i	b_i
	No	c_i	d_i

n_i

Adjusted relative incidence $= \dfrac{\Sigma\, a_i d_i / n_i}{\Sigma\, b_i c_i / n_i}$

Age < 40 years

Myocardial infarction:
Yes   No

Current oral contraceptive use:		Yes	No
	Yes	21	17
	No	26	59

47   76   123

Age 40–44 years

Myocardial infarction:
Yes   No

Current oral contraceptive use:		Yes	No
	Yes	8	2
	No	44	50

52   52   104

Adjusted relative incidence $=$
$$\frac{[(21 \times 59)/123] + [(8 \times 50)/104]}{[(17 \times 26)/123] + [(2 \times 44)/104]} = 3.14$$

for the presence or absence of heart failure. You would simply subcategorize the data according to all possible combinations of levels of the confounding factors: (a) male, mild heart failure, (b) female, mild heart failure, (c) male, no heart failure, and (d) female, no heart failure. Then, instead of calculating the adjusted rate difference (or ratio) across two subcategories, you would calculate it across four of them.

If the number of factors and/or levels becomes large, the study data may have to be spread thinly across the subcategories. The resulting adjusted difference or ratio is likely to have very wide confidence limits. To overcome this problem, one can employ one of the various forms of *multivariate analysis*. Each of these techniques postulates a mathematical model that relates the study variables to one another, and by doing so allows many separate relationships to be analyzed simultaneously. To find the type of multivariate analysis appropriate for the data you have, it is best to enlist the help of a statistician. Further general reading on the subject can be found in Rothman (1986).

REFERENCES

Colton TC: *Statistics in Medicine.* Little, Brown and Company, Boston, 1974.

Mann JI, Inman WHW: Oral contraceptives and death from myocardial infarction. *Br Med J* 1975; 2:245–248.

Mantel N, Haenszel W: Statistical aspects of the analysis of data from retrospective studies of disease. *JNCI* 1959; 22:719–748.

Rothman KJ: *Modern Perspectives in Epidemiology.* Little, Brown and Company, Boston, 1986 (in press).

Index